How to write clear medical messages

What to write and what not to write

Patrick Wulf Hanson

ACKNOWLEDGEMENTS

I have received so much valuable input, feedback and critique both before, during and after this book was completed. For this I am so very grateful.

However, I would especially like to thank four people who have provided more valuable feedback than expected.

My father, Jeremy Hanson, my English mentor and guide. You made this possible by creating a thorough interest in the English language and the importance of using it correctly. Communicating clearly in writing is an art form that comes natural to you. Thanks for sharing this.

I wish to express my most profound gratitude to my dear friend and previous colleague, Carsten Poulsen, for thorough and accurate proofreading of the manuscript. You found errors and typos that I probably couldn't even find if I specifically searched for them....

A very special thanks to Phil Leventhal for valuable feedback an encouraging me to expand the book and thereby increase the value to a broader audience.

I would not have pulled this through if it wasn't for my wonderful wife and best friend, Katja. Your accurate feedback is as valuable as your never failing support.

PATRICK WULF HANSON

CONTENTS

1 INTRODUCTION

This book was written in an attempt to provide an appropriate guide for students, young scientists and doctors who wish to improve their writing skills within the field of science and medicine.

Non-native English people communicating written medical messages will probably also find this book helpful, whereas more comprehensive textbooks are available for more experienced native English medical writers, authors, scientists and doctors.

Why do you need a writing guide? A writing guide is an important reference for many reasons. What you are reporting is probably a summary of something complicated, such as data in a report or an article, which must be clearly understood by the receiver.

Scientific writing is about communicating clinical and scientific data and information to a range of audiences in a wide variety of different formats.

Medical writers combine their knowledge of science and their research skills with an understanding of how to present information and pitch it at the right level for the intended audience.

The first secret to successfully writing about complicated subjects is to know the subject and the audience. The second secret is not to write your message in a complicated way but rather to present it as simple as possible.

As a rule, always use clear and understandable words and phrases no matter who the audience is. This applies to both formal and informal texts.

Your audience will always evaluate the content of your text based on what they understand when they read it – not necessarily what you think you have communicated!

So, instead of writing in a way that is understandable for you, make sure that you write in a way that is understandable to your audience.

Planning your communication

If you do not plan your communication rigorously, your message and its expected outcome will probably fail.

Before you start writing, think about the following five issues:

- Why do you want to communicate your message?
- What do you want to communicate, i.e. is the story worth telling?
- What do you want to show, i.e. is it interesting?
- What is the purpose of your text, i.e. what is in it for you (fame, fortune, glory)?
- To whom do you want to communicate, i.e. who is your audience?

Successful writing is also about knowing and understanding the regulatory environment to ensure that your documents are compliant with the requirements of your audience.

Writing for the pharmaceutical industry demands that you understand the industry since the rules and regulations for this type of writing are stricter and more important than in any other industry. If this is not taken seriously, forget a successful outcome of your document!

Another important aspect is to ensure a consistent use of the language. Is the preferred language of the company you are working for US English or UK English?

Although the differences are minor, there are some spelling and wording differences to consider. The style of writing also projects an image of quality regarding what you are communicating.

Never sign off a document that has not been properly proof read – there is no excuse for signing off a document that contains incorrect use of the language. It will not help your reader keep moving forward and will reflect negatively on the text, and ultimately it will reflect on you and your quality standards.

This book is a communication style guide that covers a list of topics on how to present your text based on the audience you are communicating to and it will assist you with some valuable hints while you write.

The hints include relevant grammar and spelling in medical writing, which may differ from that of other types of writing.

While every attempt has been made to ensure that the structure and content of this book reflects the principles it advocates, it is not always possible or practicable. For example, bulleted text should always have a parallel structure (for example, start with a verb in the present tense).

But this is not always the case in medical writing because one set of bulleted text may explain a concept, provide rules for implementing the concept, or provide examples of what to do or what not to do.

Terminology and rules on how to use it is explained and discussed, but it is important to always have a good English dictionary (e.g. Oxford or Cambridge dictionaries) and a medical dictionary (e.g. Dorland's or Steadman's dictionaries) at hand to check correct usage of definitions and prepositions, spelling, and hyphenation.

Many medical terms are presented in English or occasionally in Latin, depending on the target audience. As a rule, when possible, use English rather than Latin terminology.

Some medical terms are abbreviated as default whereas abbreviations as a rule should be spelled out the first time they are mentioned. Acceptable abbreviations, which would not be required to be explained, are for instance HIV and AIDS.

Finally, remember that good writing pretty much means everything that is not bad writing. Bad writing is not only poor use of words and grammar but also information that is uninteresting or presented in a confusing, unstructured manner.

In addition, bad writing is presenting incorrect or untruthful information. To ensure that your writing is good, make sure that you do your background research thoroughly.

So let us get started!

Good writing starts with knowing what you want to write. If you do not know what you want to communicate, do not communicate it. Wait until you have figured it out!

You cannot plan a good message if you have not figured out what it should be about, how it should be communicated, and to whom. Start by doing your homework about the subject, the audience and where you wish to communicate the message.

Information and sources

There are virtually thousands of websites where general information is available − Google is probably the most valuable. A specific site providing research related information is PubMed, which is a comprehensive database where most medical journals and articles are available.

More general information about diseases, conditions, symptoms and treatments can be found at sites like WebMD, Netdoctor, HNSDirect etc.

Think about how you perform your search and which keywords you use. The better keywords, the more specific and accurate information will be found.

Your audience − the stakeholder analysis

Stakeholder analysis is the technique used to identify the key people who have to be won over. You then use stakeholder management to build the support that helps you succeed. You need to rigorously address the following:

- Identify your stakeholders
- Prioritise your stakeholders
- Understand your stakeholders
  Then:
- What does your audience know?
- What does your audience need to know?
- How does your audience need to receive the message?

The stakeholder analysis is critical to the success and receipt of your message. By engaging the right people in the right way in your project, you will be able to make a big difference to its success.

As you become more skilled and successful, the actions you take and the communication projects you run will affect more and more audiences.

The more people you affect, the more likely it is that your messages will affect people who are increasingly important for your future messages and projects.

These people can become strong supporters of your work. They can also become your opponents if you do not manage them well. Draw a stakeholder grid (figure 1.) and prioritise your stakeholders.

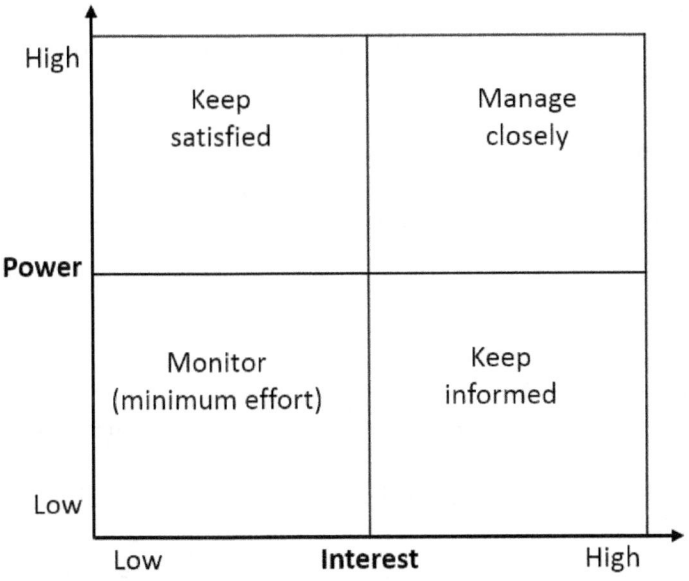

Figure 1. Prioritise your stakeholders by adding their names where you think they belong in the stakeholder prioritising grid.

A thorough stakeholder analysis and the subsequent stakeholder management is an important process that successful people use to win support from others.

Prioritise it, dedicate lots of time to it, and learn how to do it really well. It will help you ensure that your projects succeed where others fail.

Interviewing sources

Stakeholders are usually important people who are responsible for promoting research, a company, a hospital etc. Stakeholders may help you identify opportunities, products or processes that could influence your target audience.

Most stakeholders will immediately view you as an allied, whereas some will inevitably view you as a threat rather than helpful. When you talk about doing research and fulfilling some of the requirements, you may be treading on territory they view as theirs.

If you are pushing a view that is not the same as theirs, you have the potential to make them look bad. Choose your questions wisely and ask the questions that your stakeholder is best equipped to answer.

Consider the following

- Make sure that your questions are not vague, i.e. your questions must be specific
- Prepare to rephrase your questions if you do not get the answer you expect
- Your questions should be open-ended. Ask "what do you think about…", where the interviewee will express what he thinks instead of asking "do you agree about…", where the interviewee can answer "yes" or "no"
- Avoid leading questions since they may lead to non-committing answers
- Make sure that the order of your questions is logical, i.e. each question and answer should lead to the next question.

Now contact the interviewee and make an appointment for the interview.

2 WRITING AS A COMMUNICATION TOOL

Language, grammar and spelling

Choosing the correct way of writing something may not necessarily be the right way. The right way is, however, always the correct way! If you write solely for you, and you are your own audience, this is irrelevant.

But most writers are communicating their content to others. Understanding what your target audience knows, what they do not know and what they need to know is what will help you present the text in the best possible way.

It is easy to communicate something complicated, but it is a lot more difficult to communicate it so that it is understood.

The greatest challenge is to communicate something that is not only understood but also has a desired effect in your audience. So, keeping the text as short and simple as possible is good, but not always right.

When you present something complicated, your message may be very short and simple, to be communicated to a well-informed audience that understands the subject clearly (e.g. to doctors), the same message may need a lot more explaining to other audiences (e.g. to patients).

Active voice

As a general rule always use an active voice unless you specifically want a passive sentence. The active voice is used to indicate that the grammatical subject of the verb is performing the action or causing the happening denoted by the verb.

An example of active voice is "the girl threw the ball" whereas in passive voice "the ball was thrown by the girl". The word "by" is often an indication that the passive voice is being used.

A brief brush-up of grammar, words and their use

Verbs

The verb is perhaps the most important part of the sentence. A verb or compound verb asserts something about the subject of the sentence and expresses actions, events, or states of being. The verb or compound verb is the critical element of the predicate of a sentence.

The pattern of a simple sentence is largely determined by the type of verb it contains. There are three verb types: intransitive, linking and transitive.

Intransitive verbs

An intransitive verb can occur alone in the predicate of a sentence, because it requires no other sentence element to complete its meaning (for example, "John complained", "the rain poured", "the patient smiled").

Linking verbs

The common linking verb "be" does not denote any kind of action, unlike other verbs (for example, "run", "shout", "drink", "snore").

Instead, the linking verb links the subject to another word following the verb (for example, "John looks healthy", "the patient seems happy", "Mrs Anderson looks pale").

Transitive verbs

A transitive verb requires another sentence element to complete its meaning, and cannot stand alone in the predicate of a sentence.

For example, use the verb "create", which is a verb that needs something following it, since you must create something (for example, "Picasso created art", "the saint created miracles", "the professor creates a good atmosphere").

A verb usually has 5 different forms:

Base form:	the doctor decided to treat the patient
The -s form:	the doctor treats the patient
Past form:	the doctor treated the patient
The -ed form:	the doctor has treated the patient
The -ing form:	the doctor is treating the patient

In regular verbs, two of the forms are identical: the past form ("treated") and the -ed form ("treated"). However, these two forms are not always identical:

Base form:	the doctor will write a prescription
The -s form:	the doctor writes a prescription
Past form:	the doctor wrote a prescription
The -ed form:	the doctor has written a prescription
The -ing form:	the doctor is writing a prescription

A verb thus expresses existence, action, or occurrence in most languages. If it is possible, try to replace a noun phrase with a verb (for example, replace "his speech indicated that" with "he said" or "he implied").

This makes the message clearer.

Replace weak verbs (for example, get, be, do, go, become) with stronger, more specific ones whenever possible (for example, write "Dr Smith received the results" not "Dr Smith got the results").

This will strengthen the communicated message.

Ensure that the subject of sentences that begin "There is...", "There are...", or "It is..." are not ambiguous.

If there is any ambiguity, rewrite the sentence. Confusing, conflicting or bad sentences result in lowering the quality of the document. For example, "the patient had an adverse event" not "the patient experienced an adverse event".

Be

The verb "be" is very irregular, and exhibits a total of eight different forms:

Base form: be
Present form: am, are, is
Past form: was, were
The -ed form: been
The -ing form: being

Subject and predicate

The subject is the noun, noun phrase, or pronoun in a sentence or clause that denotes the doer of the action or what is described by the predicate.

The predicate modifies the subject and includes the verb, objects or phrases governed by the verb. Examples: "opened the door" in "Mark opened the door" or "is very sleepy" in "The child is very sleepy".

Ensure that your sentences are properly built up by identifying the subject and predicate.

The subject thus is the person or procedure that is being discussed or described (for example, "treatment") whereas the predicate is the part of a statement that says something about the subject (for example, "is necessary" in "treatment is necessary").

Always try to use a singular predicate when "with", "together with", "including", "as well as", "no less than", or "plus" between the subject and predicate is used (for example, "Bonny, together with Clyde, is presenting the new product").

Use a singular predicate for two singular nouns joined using "or" or "nor" (for example, "Bonny or Clyde is presenting the product").

A plural predicate is used for two nouns by joining "and" (for example, "Bonny and Clyde are presenting the new product"). When a plural noun and a singular noun are joined using "or" or "nor", the predicate agrees with the closest noun: "Clyde or the guests were to pay the bill". "The guests or Clyde was to pay the bill"

Use a singular predicate for organisations because they are single entities and should be treated as singular (for example, "The board is", "the group is", "Apple Inc. is").

Use a singular predicate for constructions such as: "The auditor, Anderson, McCarthy and Smith Partners…". "Anderson, McCarthy and Smith Partners, auditor for the study…"

None – singular or plural?

Use the noun that follows "none" to determine whether "none" is singular or plural (for example, "None of the alcohol was wasted", "None of the explanations are valid").

None is widely used as the equivalent to no one, and therefore requires a singular verb and singular pronoun (for example, "None of the players was given a drink".

However, write "none" if you mean "zero", not "not one". For example, write "none of the dishes tasted good", instead of "not one of the dishes tasted good", since "not one" may lead to confusion because it can mean "zero" or "any number greater than one".

Tense and indirect speech

Always use the past tense when your source talks about something that is happening at the time of the conversation (for example, "Dr Anderson said the new drug was producing great results.").

Use the past perfect tense when your source talks about something that happened before the interview (for example, "Dr Anderson said the new drug had not been available last year").

Use the conditional tense when your source talks about something that is happening in the future (for example, "Dr Brown said the new drug would not be available until next year").

Use the same tense chosen by the speaker when you write "according to" sentences (for example, "The new drug will not be available this year", according to Dr Anderson.).

Do not use "that" when attributing indirect speech (unless the sentence is ambiguous without it) (for example, write "She said she would attend the conference" not "She said that she would attend the conference").

Use "that" when attributing indirect speech if the sentence is ambiguous without it (for example, "She said yesterday she would attend the conference" to distinguish it from "She said that yesterday she would attend the conference").

Participles

Misplaced participles (or dangling modifiers) can cause confusion (for example, "Being in a wrecked condition, I was able to buy the house very cheap").

In this example, the modifier (the phrase that describes a person or thing) does not modify the correct noun. This confusion usually requires the sentence to be rewritten.

Contractions

Always spell out words properly and omit from using contractions of verbs in print unless quoting direct speech, and then use an apostrophe (for example, I'll [I will], won't [will not], they're [they are], didn't [did not], can't [cannot], let's [let us], it's [it is]).

Contractions of some nouns no longer use the apostrophe (for example, phone [telephone], flu [influenza]).

Verbal nouns

Some nouns have become verbs ("shop" became "to shop", "ship" became "to ship") and others are becoming accepted ("to lunch", "to video"). Do not assume the process is automatic, do not use "to impact".

Nouns

A noun is a word used to name a person, animal, place, thing, and abstract idea. Nouns are usually the first words which small children learn.

Most nouns can be identified by their endings (for example, "-ence", "-ment", "-ism", "-tion"), and most nouns have a singular and a plural form.

The nouns will change from singular to plural by adding "-s" (for example, "scalpel – scalpels", "syringe – syringes", "doctor – doctors").

However, some nouns have irregular plurals (for example, "woman – women", "man – men", "mouse – mice", foot – feet").

Never change verbs to nouns, and do not change nouns to verbs (for example, write "we can reuse these data in the next calculation" not "we can leverage these data in the next calculation").

Sometimes a noun describes another noun. In that case the noun acts like an adjective (for example, "a bicycle shop", were bicycle acts as an adjective).

Do not use nouns as adjectives unless they are in singular form (for example, "a bicycles shop" or "brush your teeth with a teethbrush" are incorrect. Sentences filled with noun phrases are typically easier to read when broken into two simpler sentences.

Prepositions

Correct and exact use of prepositions strengthens writing; it may be better to use "within", "inside", or "into", than to use "in" for all situations.

Plurals

The plural is usually formed by adding "s" to the word or abbreviation (without an apostrophe) (for example, "hospital" becomes "hospitals", "event" becomes "events").

For a Greek-derived word that ends in "on", replace "on" with "a" (for example, "criterion" becomes "criteria"), or add "s" (for example, "skeleton" becomes "skeletons"). For a Greek-derived word that ends in "pus", add "es" (for example, "octopus" becomes "octopuses").

For a Latin-derived word that ends in "us", add "es" (for example, "status" becomes "statuses"), or replace "us" with "era" (for example, "genus" becomes "genera").

However, the plural "s" does not apply to abbreviated units (for example, 20 km [not kms], 45 g [not gs], 2.3 kg, 30 cl). The plural of "curriculum vitae" is "curricula vitae", "information is", "the criterion is", "the media are", "the data are".

Never use an apostrophe before years to indicate a decade (for example, write "the research paper was written in the 1990s" not "the research paper was written in the '90's").

Possessives

The possessive is formed using an apostrophe (') sometimes followed by "s":

- For singular nouns, add "'s" (for example, "a patient's result").
- For singular nouns that end in "s", add only the apostrophe (for example, "thrombosis' effects").
- For singular nouns that end in "ss", add "'s" (for example, "the boss's comments").
- For plural nouns that do not end in "s", add "'s" (for example, "women's rights").
- For plural nouns that end in "s", add only the apostrophe (for example, "three patients' results").
- For names that end in "s", add "'s" (for example, "she was in Dr Williams's office").
- For plurals of names that end in "s", make the plural and add the apostrophe (for example, "the Joneses' dinner party was successful").
- For nouns related to time, add "'s" (for example, "today's meeting", "yesterday's discussion", "last year's conference").
- Use the construction "10 years of treatment" not "10 years' treatment".

Organisations and institutions often omit the apostrophe, but always check (for example, "Junior Doctors Association", but "Chiropractic Doctor's Association of Stockholm").

Never use an apostrophe with possessive pronouns (for example, his, hers, theirs, ours, yours, its). Note the difference between "Assessments are made on Fridays [plural – no apostrophe] during the study" and "This Friday's [possessive] assessment will be in the new offices."

Adjectives

An adjective modifies a noun or a pronoun by describing, identifying, or quantifying words. An adjective usually precedes the noun or the pronoun which it modifies (for example, "a hungry patient", "a sick patient", "a clean wound").

Most adjectives can end with "-ble", "-ive", "-ous", "-y", and occur before a noun (active voice) or after a linking verb (passive voice).

The base adjective form "sick" has two other forms, i.e. "sicker" (the comparative form) and "sickest" (the superlative form).

The comparative form is produced by adding an -er ending, and the superlative form is produced by adding an -est ending, to the base form. The words "good" and "bad" are irregular adjectives ("Good, better, best" and "bad, worse, worst").

Adverbs

An adverb can modify a verb, an adjective, another adverb, a phrase, or a clause. An adverb indicates manner, time, place, cause, or degree and answers questions such as "how," "when," "where," "how much".

Some adverbs can be identified by their characteristic "ly" suffix (for example, "caring – caringly", "slow – slowly", "soft – softly"), but most of them must be identified by untangling the grammatical relationships within the sentence or clause as a whole.

Unlike an adjective, an adverb can be found in various places within the sentence and have no distinctive ending (for example, "soon", "today", "tomorrow", "yesterday", "now").

Pronouns

A pronoun can replace a noun or another pronoun that has already been or is about to be used in the sentence or context. You use pronouns like "he", "which," "none," and "you" to make your sentences less cumbersome and less repetitive. The major subclasses of pronouns are personal, possessive and reflexive.

Personal pronoun

A personal pronoun refers to a specific person or thing and changes its form to indicate person, number, gender, and case (for example, "he", "him", "I", "you", "she", "it", "we", "you", "they").

Possessive pronoun

A possessive pronoun indicates that the pronoun is acting as a marker of possession and defines who owns a particular object or person (for example, "mine", "yours", "hers", "his", "its", "ours", "theirs").

Note that possessive pronouns are very similar to possessive adjectives like "my", "her", and "their".

Reflexive pronoun

A reflexive pronoun is used to refer back to the subject of the clause or sentence (for example, "myself", "yourself", "herself", "himself", "itself", "ourselves", "yourselves", "themselves").

Prepositions

A preposition links nouns, pronouns and phrases to other words in a sentence. The word or phrase that the preposition introduces is called the object of the preposition.

A preposition usually indicates the temporal, spatial or logical relationship of its object to the rest of the sentence (for example, "after", "around", "before").

Conjunctions

Conjunctions are used to link individual words, phrases and clauses together (for example, "and", "but", "or", "nor", "for", "so", "yet").

Punctuations

Commas

In British English, a comma is not usually used with and between the two last items in a series or list (e.g. Days 1, 2 and 5) whereas in American English a comma is used (Days 1, 2, and 5).

Place a comma after adverbial and prepositional clauses initiating a sentence (for example, "As of 1 October 2005, 17 subjects were enrolled").

Use commas in compound sentences (for example, "The queen decided to stay in for the evening, but she did not watch television").

Use commas to set off non-restrictive clauses (for example, "The lawnmower, which is broken anyway, hasn't been used in years").

Use commas to separate elements in a series, and use a comma before the conjunction in a simple series (for example, write "the packaging is red, white, and blue", not "the packaging is red, white and blue").

Use a comma before the concluding conjunction in a series if an integral element of the series requires a conjunction (for example, write "We invited representatives from marketing, sales, and research and development to the meeting", not "We invited representatives from marketing, sales and research and development to the meeting.").

Use commas to separate a series of adjectives equal in rank. If the commas can be replaced using the word "and" without changing the meaning, the adjectives are equal (for example, "a simple, precise measurement", "a popular, effective treatment").

Do not use a comma when the last adjective before a noun outranks its predecessors – it is then an integral element of a noun phrase, which is grammatically equivalent to a single noun (for example, write "a successful clinical trial", not "a successful, clinical trial" – the noun phrase is "clinical trial").

Use a comma to separate an introductory clause or phrase from a main clause (for example, "When the nausea ended, she increased the dose"). The comma may be omitted after short introductory phrases if no ambiguity results (for example, "During the study there were many successes.").

Use a comma if its omission causes misunderstanding (for example, "Before eating, the patient took the tablet"). Use a comma before the conjunction in most cases.

A conjunction (for example, and, but, or) links two clauses that could stand alone as separate sentences (for example, "He was depressed at the start of the study, but the treatment worked for him.").

Use a comma if the subject of each clause is expressly stated (for example, "We are attending the congress in Stockholm in the spring, and we plan to launch the drug in the autumn").

Do not use a comma when the subject of the two clauses is the same and is not repeated in the second (for example, "We are visiting Stockholm and will visit the old town").

Use commas around addresses and titles in the text (for example, "the samples were analysed in Laboratory X, Amsterdam, and then shipped to England", "the investigator, M Johnson, PhD, screened all the patients").

Use a comma to separate information without losing the meaning of the sentence (for example, "Drug Inc's new product, Aspirin, will help patients with headache", "Aspirin, a new product from Drug Inc, will help patients with headache").

Colons

Colons are used to introduce that something follows like an example, quotation or a list. In general text, do not capitalise words that follow a colon. However, in headings and titles, do capitalise after a colon (for example,"Humira: The biologic treatment against rheumatoid arthritis.").

If only one sentence follows the colon, do not capitalise the first word of the new sentence. If two or more sentences follow the colon, capitalise the first word of each sentence following (for example, "I enjoy reading: it beats watching the clock", "Garlic is used in Italian cooking: It greatly enhances the flavour of pasta dishes. It also enhances the flavour of the pizza").

The colon replaces words like "includes" or "including". In many cases, it should be thought of as an equals sign (=), in that the items on one side of the colon are equal to the description on the other side (for example, "Lemonade has three basic ingredients: lemon juice, water and lots of sugar").

Semicolons

Semicolons are used to join two independent clauses, to separate main clauses joined by a conjunctive adverb or to separate things in a list that are already separated with commas.

It is not always clear whether a colon or a semicolon suits your purpose. The semicolon is usually used to link independent clauses not joined by a coordinating conjunction. Semicolons should join only those independent clauses that are closely related in meaning.

Semicolons always join two complete sentences, which is not necessarily the case for colons, especially when introducing a list (for example, "When it comes to asking friends for money, I have one word of advice: don't".

In some cases, either will do nicely. Keep the following in mind when you use a semicolon:

- Each clause should be complete, containing both subject and verb
- The two clauses should be closely related in meaning
- Do not capitalise the word that follows the semicolon unless that word is a proper noun
- Limit your use of semicolons.

Semicolons are like glasses of champagne; save them for special occasions. Semicolons should also be used in cases of long and very complex lists.

In such lists, a semicolon may be used before "and", which is different from the normal list-comma rule (for example, "John had to make sure his suitcase was packed, given that he would leave directly from work; check that all his tasks were done, even the assignments not due until next week; check that he had the phone numbers of his uncle, both sets of grandparents and his one cousin, because he would have no way to contact them once he was in transit, and he didn't want to be stranded; and remember to water the plants, feed the cat and close all windows in the house before he left in the morning."").

Apostrophe

Apostrophes indicate ownership (for example, "the patient's") or a contraction (for example, "didn't"). You should use an apostrophe to form the possessive case of a noun or to show that you have left out letters in a contraction (for example, "it's" ["i" in "it is"], so it's a contraction like "didn't").

Brackets

Round brackets "( )", or parentheses, are used to include useful information in the sentence, without slowing the flow. For example, "The patient was late (by more than 2 hours), but we waited.".

Use square brackets "[ ]" to insert brackets within parenthesis, or to insert a comment (for example, "The patient (who was late [due to heavy traffic]) indicated no sign of headache.").

Dash

A dash is similar to a hyphen or minus sign but it differs from both of these symbols primarily in length and function. The most common versions of the dash are the en dash (–) and the longer em dash (—). A dash can be used at the beginning and end of parenthetical information.

Usually, you will use dashes when you want to emphasise the information, but you might also use them if the parenthetical information is too long or abrupt to be set off with commas.

The en dash "–" is often used instead of a colon, although they are not always interchangeable (for example, "Six doctors attended – all of them surgeons"). Always leave a space on either side of an en dash.

Ellipsis

Use an ellipsis (three full stops) to indicate missing words in a quoted passage. MS Word auto-formats three full stops to an ellipsis, if not otherwise specified.

If the ellipsis is not auto-formatted, add a space before and after each of the three full stops (for example, "The FDA ensures... public health protection.").

An ellipsis (for example, when the last part of a quoted sentence is omitted) at the end of a sentence with no subsequent sentence should be followed with a space and a period, i.e. a total of four full stops (for example, "...some depression scales...").

End punctuation

The punctuation marks the end of a sentence, and can be the period, the question mark and the exclamation mark. The period that terminates a sentence is by far the most common of the end punctuation marks.

You may also use periods with imperative sentences that have no sense of urgency or excitement attached. Do not use to separate or after the initials of people's names (for example, WC Fields [no space between initials]).

Do not use full stop after abbreviations, degrees, titles, or units of measure (for example, BSc, PhD, Ms, Dr, St, Ave, Co, Ltd, km, g, the Rev).

Do not use end punctuation between or after the letters in abbreviations of organisations, states, countries (for example, BMA, NY, UK, US), or chemicals (for example, DDT, 2, 4,5-T, PVC, TNT).

When you want to express a sense of urgency or very strong emotion, you may end your imperative sentences and statements with an exclamation mark, and use a question mark at the end of a direct question.

Hyphen

Only hyphenate individual words in tables. Hyphenate compound adjectives (for example, "ibuprofen-treated patients" and "flexible-dose study").

Hyphenate an implied noun (for example, "When she was a sixty-year-old [woman]"), but do not hyphenate a compound adjective if it is not ambiguous (for example, "When she was sixty years old").

Use more than one hyphen if necessary (for example, "up-to-date figures").

Use a nonbreaking hyphen between words that should not break (for example, "SK 197-017").

Hyphenate adverbial compounds that do not end in "-ly" when they are a part of the subject (for example, "a well-known reason", "a well-tolerated drug"), but do not hyphenate when they are a part of the predicate (for example, "the reason is well known", "the drug is well tolerated").

Hyphenate adjectival forms that end in "-ly" (for example, "silly-looking arrangement"). Do not hyphenate adverbial compounds that end in "-ly" (for example, write "wholly owned subsidiary", not "wholly-owned subsidiary").

Do not hyphenate individual words in running text, particularly 'align left' text. 'Align left' text is text that is lined up with the left side of the margin, and is also known as 'left justified' text.

Do not use the "-ed" ending if it can be removed (for example, "three-arm study", "nine-hole golf course"). Note that the word "group" is preferred to "arm".

Do not hyphenate most prefixes and the word stem, even if the same letter adjoins (for example, "reenter", "coordinate").

Do not use complex constructions (for example, "the old hair-of-the-dog-that-bit-you remedy").

Hyphenated words

Many words are hyphenated as a noun (for example, "read-out"), but not as a verb (for example, "read out").

If you can insert another word between the two words, then it is not hyphenated (for example, "read it out"). Check that you are using hyphens correctly in proper nouns.

Punctuation in tables

Do not use ditto marks (") for repeated items; supply the numbers. Use an en dash (–) to indicate entries that are not supplied or not applicable; do not use "NA" or "n/a". If more explanation is required, add a footnote to the en dash (for example, "–a") and write the explanation under the table. Use "0" to indicate that data were available and had a value of zero.

Quotation marks

Quotation marks have several functions:

- They indicate exactly what has been said or written by a person
- They indicate words used in a special way (for example, a "so-called" adverse event)
- They indicate some titles (for example, article and symposia titles in text, but not in the reference list)
- They indicate familiar names (for example, Elvis "The King" Presley)
- Use double quotation marks in all cases, except inside double quotation marks (for example, "He discussed the 'so-called' adverse events in the article," she said.)
- Italics are preferred for special terms (names of books, magazines, journals, films, and plays should be italicised).

Slash or stroke (/)

It is also called an oblique, diagonal, separatrix, virgule, scratch comma, slant, or forward slash (it is similar to a solidus [or shilling mark], which is a separate punctuation mark).

Add a space on either side of a slash in quoting multiple lines from a headline, poem, or play.

Add a thin space in FrameMaker and no space in Word on either side of a slash when used to replace "or" in "he/she" or "his/her".

Do not add a space at any other time (including units and computer language). Use "and/or" only if absolutely necessary; "or" is almost always sufficient.

Do not use a slash in text as a symbol for "or", or "and" (for example, write "indexing or abstracting", not "indexing/abstracting").

Do not use a slash in text as a symbol for "per" (except for units such as "mg/day").

Attribution

Statements and comments must be attributed to the person who made them. Facts must be attributed to their source, unless they are absolutely a matter of common knowledge (for example, "The earth revolves around the sun.").

Bullets

Use parallel structure in bulleted text. Use bullets to indicate that items in a list are separate and in no particular order. Begin each new entry with a left-justified bullet and double-check alphabetical lists to ensure the correct order.

Use lowercase, do not include "and" in the list, and do not use punctuation at the end of each bullet point, unless each is a complete sentence. For example, "The orchards were filled with:
- apples
- pears
- plums".

Credit line

Include credit for a photograph or illustration immediately below the photograph or illustration and just above the caption (for example, "photograph by Geir Haukurson").

Acknowledge a table of data drawn from another source in a footnote to the table. Do not include a credit line for illustrations or tables made by the author.

Figures (Illustrations)

Use a non-breaking space between "Figure" and the number (for example, "Figure 1"). Use "Figure 1" to refer to a figure referred to in the text (for example, write "...is illustrated in Figure 1 [object]", not "Figure 1 [subject] illustrates..."). Use "(Figure 1)" to refer to a figure not referenced in the text (for example, "...increase in the number of remitters (Figure 1)").

Do not refer to the figure's position (for example, write "...is illustrated in

Figure 1.", not "...is shown in Figure 1, below."). Do not use "see" (for example, "see Figure 1").

Footnotes

Use footnotes in tables only; do not use them in running text. Use alphabetic footnote indicators: a, b, c, d, and so on. Use an en dash (–) to indicate entries that are not supplied or not applicable in a table.

If more explanation is required, add a footnote (for example, "–a") and write the explanation under the table. Do not use numeric footnote indicators.

Do not use * as a footnote indicator (unless it means statistical significance). Do not have the footnote hyperlinked (blue font and underlined), it must be a black font and not underlined.

Page references

Use a non-breaking space between "page" and the number (for example, "page 54"). Page references should always be lower case "page". In most cases, the page references will be in parentheses (for example, "(page 54)").

In clinical study reports, never refer to a narrative using its specific page number; refer to the narratives' section (for example, write "For further details, refer to narratives of deaths, other serious adverse events, withdrawals due to adverse events, and other significant adverse events on page 543.").

Running text

Running text consists of paragraphs, bulleted and numbered lists, and hanging indents or definition lists.

Splitting words is not normally necessary as we do not hyphenate or justify text in running text.

In posters and very narrow columns in tables, you may need to split the occasional word using a hyphen.

If possible, do not break proper names. However, if a proper name has to be broken, break between the elements (for example, write" Steve Ball-mer", not "Steve Bal-lmer").

Spelling

There are several areas where spelling differ between British and American English.

If it is not predefined, e.g. in instructions for authors (medical journals) it is wise to find out if your audience is American, British, Australian etc.

If your message is intended for a wider, unspecific English audience, the most important issue is to be consistent. Either stick to the British or the American English spelling.

My general rule is if American English is not specified choose British English. Most scientific journals require British English.

When a dictionary provides more than one way of spelling a word, use the first option, unless a specific style guide you are following says otherwise.

British vs. American English

If you choose to use British English, be consequent and avoid Americanisms (British/American): lift/elevator, holiday/vacation, fall/autumn, lavatory/restroom, etc.

In constructions such as "2 am Friday", use "2 am on Friday".

Note that some spelling differs:

- Words that end in "our/or" (British vs. American): "behaviour" versus "behavior"

- Words that end in "ise/ize" (British vs. American): "capitalise" versus "capitalize".

In general, use English medical terms instead of American or Latin medical terms.

Note the spelling for the following words:

British English	American English
Aluminium	Aluminum
Analyse	Analyze
Catalogue	Catalog
Centre	Center
Cheque (from a bank)	check
colour	Color
Defence	Defense
Honour	Honor
Foetus	Fetus
Haemophilia	Hemophilia
hyperglycaemia	Hyperglycemia
Labour	Labor
Metre	Meter
Oedema	Edema
Oestrogen	Estrogen
Pyjamas	Pajamas
Paralyse	Paralyze
Practise (verb)	Practice
Programme (unless it is a computer program)	program
Theatre	Theater
Whisky	Whiskey (Both American and Irish)

Ensure your computer's spell-checker is set to "English (British)" or "English (US)", depending on your target audience. This book follows the British spelling.

Review your text carefully since spell-checkers are unable to detect incorrect homonyms ("there", "they're", "their") or usage ("form", "from").

3 MEANING AND USE OF WORDS

Accommodation and accomodation

Accommodation (with double m) is the act of accommodating or the state of being accommodated, whereas accomodation (with a single m) is the process by which the eye adapts to maintain a clear and focused image on an object as the distance to the object varies.

Advice or advise

Advice is a noun, which means that you are offered an opinion from someone about what or how you should do something in a specific situation.

Advice is an uncountable noun and is therefore always singular (for example, "I would like you to give me some advice.").

Advise is a verb, which means to provide information and suggest specific types of action (for example, "I advise you to listen to your doctor.").

Alot

Do not use "alot". Use "a lot" or "a large amount", because of the potential confusion between "a lot" and the related verb "allot" (which means "assign").

Alright or all right

Even though it is not incorrect to use "alright", use "all right" (for example, "the patient told them he would be all right"). Mergers such as altogether and already are fully acceptable, whereas alright is currently considered to be accepted by Microsoft's spell-checker, I still recommend to use "all right".

Amongst, amidst, and whilst

Always use the simpler "among", "amid", "while" and do not use the more old-fashioned "whilst", "amongst", "amidst", "unbeknownst" and "albeit".

And and or, neither and nor

When distinguishing between two things, only use "nor" after "neither" (for example, "it was neither one thing nor the other").

In negative constructions ("no", "not", "none"), "or" rather than "and" is usually correct (for example, "the patient was not permitted to take aspirin, paracetamol, or ibuprofen during the study").

If "and" were used, then the patient was not permitted to take the combination, but each drug separately was permitted. In negative constructions, "neither" and "nor" are rarely correct as they lead to double negation (for example, "the patient did not attend neither the first nor the second visit" means the patient did attend the visits).

Anticipate or expect

The two words are often used as synonyms but in formal use "anticipate" implies a more concrete prediction than "expect", i.e. to feel or realise beforehand, or to foresee something making you more likely to react since you know that you will need to.

Expect, however, is to regard something as probable or likely, i.e. you predict something (for example, "the young doctor expected the patient to be discharged after two days, whereas the more experienced consultant anticipated that the patient would need at least another day to recover").

Anytime, Anymore, Anyday

Use "any time", "any more", "any day. Do not use "anytime", "anymore" and "anyday". The two-word version "any time" is a noun phrase that means "any amount of time" or "any particular time".

The single word "anytime" is an adverb (which modifies a verb), and therefore means "whenever", "on any occasion" or "at any time".

Breech and breach

The" breech" is the lower rear portion of the human trunk, i.e. the buttocks, while the "breach" refers to an action taken by someone in an agreement, for example, "breach of confidence".

By and using

The word "using" is often more correct than "by" – "using" should be used for methodology, "by" should be used for people. For example, write:

- "the data were analysed using regression analysis" not "the data were analysed by regression analysis"
- "the data were analysed by a statistician".

Common sense and common-sense

"Common sense" is a noun (for example, "it is common sense to keep medicine from children") whereas "common-sense" is an adjectival construction (for example, "he admired her common-sense approach to problems").

Comparisons

Always use "different from" (for example, "...was different from that anticipated.") or "different to" (for example, "...different to previous studies.").

Do not use "different than". Use "compared with" or "compared to". Do not use "2-fold increase". Use "doubled" or "changed by a factor of 2".

Do not use "a number of". Instead, use "several". Use "-er" when comparing 2 things (for example, "this effect is bigger than that effect").

Use "-est" when comparing 3 or more things (for example, "this effect is the biggest we have seen with this product").

Complementary or complimentary

"Complementary" serves to fill out or complete something else, i.e. it completes something, while "complimentary" is an expression of praise, congratulation or encouragement (for example, "a complimentary drink" refers to a free drink.

Counsel or council

To "counsel" someone means providing advice (e.g. by a counsellor), whereas a "council" is an assembly of people called together for consultation, deliberation, or discussion.

The council is often gathered to agree, decide or suggest something.

Dependent or dependant

"Dependent" means relying on or requiring the aid for support, i.e. being dependent of something (for example, "the patient is insulin dependent", and an example of the opposite is, "the insulin pump works independently").

A "dependant" is someone who is dependent of something, i.e. he/she depends on another person, organisation, etc., for support or aid.

Discreet or discrete

"Discreet" means showing prudence and self-restraint in speech and behaviour (for example, "he discreetly asked for a second opinion"). "Discrete" means that something is separate or distinct.

In or into

"In" is generally used when describing the position of something (for example, "the blood is in the vein"), while "into" is describes the direction (for example, "the drug was injected into the vein").

It's or its

"It's" is a shortening of "it is" (for example, "it's time for surgery"), while "its" is the possessive form if "it" (for example, "he inspected the wound and cleaned its surrounding").

Lead or led

To "lead" is to show the way by going in front ("the experienced consultant will lead the young doctors through the procedure"), whereas "led" is the past particle of lead (for example, "the experienced consultant led the young doctors through the procedure").

Licence and License

"Licence" is a noun and means an official document (for example, "this drug has a licence from the authorities"), whereas "license" is a verb and means to give a licence to somebody (for example, "the manufacturer asked the authorities to license their new drug").

Meiosis or miosis

"Meiosis" is a type of cell division in which a nucleus divides into four daughter nuclei, each containing half the chromosome number of the parent nucleus in sexually reproducing organisms. "Miosis" is the constriction of the pupil of the eye, resulting from a normal response to an increase in light. It can also be caused by certain drugs or pathological conditions.

Per cent, Percentage, and Proportion

"Per cent" is parts per hundred. Write "per cent" (not the American "percent") only at the beginning of a sentence (for example, "Sixty-six per cent of patients reached full remission."). Write "%" for a specific number and only with numerals (for example, ". . . the final 5%."). "Percentage" is the number, amount, or rate of something, expressed per 100.

"Proportion" is a part or share of a whole (for examples, "The proportion of regular smokers increases with age.", "A higher proportion of Americans than Britons are prescribed antibiotics.").

Proportion can also be the relationship (ratio) of one thing to another in size or amount (for example, "The proportion of men to women with pneumonia has changed over the years."). Use "proportion" not "percentage" in text.

Practice and Practise

"Practice" is a noun referring to a place (for example, "He visited the doctor's practice."), whereas "practise" is a verb referring to an act (for example, "Dr Anderson practises medicine in Stockholm.").

Prescribe or proscribe

To "prescribe" is to give specific directions, either orally or in writing, for the preparation and administration of medicine to be used in the treatment of a medical condition. "Proscribe", however, is to prohibit or forbid something.

Principle or principal

"Principle" refers the moral or ethical standards, or judgements in a person (for instance, "the doctor is a man of principle"), whereas a "principal" is the first, highest, or number one in importance, rank, worth, or degree (a principal is another word for a school headmaster or dean).

Sometimes, some time, some times, sometime

These all have separate, distinct meanings and are not interchangeable (for examples, "I fish sometimes.", "I will go fishing at some time.", "Some times are better for fishing than others.", "I'm a sometime [former] fisherman."

That and which

"That" and "which" are relative pronouns and are not interchangeable – "which" is not the literary form of "that".

Use "that" in restricted clauses not preceded by a comma (for example, "The house that Jack built is still standing").

Use "which" and commas in unrestricted clauses (for example, "The house, which Jack built, is still standing").

Further explanation: The first example is restricted to one particular house whereas the second is not restricted, i.e. it may indicate that it is merely one of the houses that Jack built.

The clause between the commas simply adds extra information that is not essential to the sentence.

Volume and quantity

Always use "fewer" (instead of "less") with numbers of individual items or people (for example, "There were fewer patients in Group A.").

Use "less than" for quantity measures (for example, "less than 700 tonnes of tablets", "less than 200 pounds").

"More than/less than" and "over/under" are not interchangeable (for example, "There are more than [not over] 30 people in the room", "The book costs less than €12."). Do not use "over" to express a period of time.

Non-native English speakers generally understand the phrase "The study extends over 2 years" to mean longer than 2 years. In this example, "over" means to "during" a period of time. It does thus not mean that the study extended "more than" 2 years.

The word "both" only applies when two items are included (for example, write "Both paracetamol and ibuprofen" not "Both paracetamol, ibuprofen and placebo.").

Use "both… and" to emphasise that one is talking of two separate things (for example, "both in the safety and in the efficacy analyses"). Incorrect placement or incautious use of "both" can lead to misunderstanding (for example, "both patients and subjects" could mean "2 [specific] patients and subjects").

Usage of words

Age

Write the age between commas (for example, "John Smith, aged 25 years, explained") or as a compound adjective (for example, "The patient, a 25-year-old man, explained...").

In a feature article, present the information in the best way (for example, "a researcher in his twenties"). To stress age, highlight it (for example, "a 25-year-old researcher made this discovery").

Believe

Report what people say and not what you believe they are thinking (for example, write "Dr Jones said he believed the results were correct", not "Dr Jones believes the results were correct" – you do not know what he was thinking).

Dimensions

Write "m²", not "sq m" (for "square meter"). Use the multiplication symbol (×) in measurements (for example, "2½ × 6-metre room"), not the letter 'x'.

Disc and Disk

Write "disk" for a computer disk (for example, "hard disk", "floppy disk").

Write "disc" for other flat, round objects (for example, "compact disc", "intervertebral disc").

E-mail Addresses

Write e-mail addresses in lowercase (for example, information@information.com).

Euphemism

A euphemism is a gentler word than the one normally used to refer to something unpleasant. Do not use euphemisms (for example, write "died", not the euphemism "passed away").

Fractions

Use text and hyphens for amounts less than one in text (for example, write "one-third of the patients were men", not "⅓ of the patients..."). Use numerals for amounts greater than one (for example, 1⅔, 2⅝). Use keyboard symbols (for example, symbol "½" and do not type "1/2").

Only use proper fractions (a fraction with a numerator [top number] less than its denominator [bottom number]) (for example, write "1⅔", not "5/3").

Avoid denominators greater than 4 (for example, "two-ninths"). Instead, use decimals or per cent (for example, "0.22" or "62.5%"). Use a colon with ratios given with numerals (for example, "the ratio of women to men was 2:1").

Gender versus sex

Use the word "sex", not "gender". Use the nouns "man" and "woman" for people, and "male" and "female" for animals.

Do not use male terms generically; use "spokesman" and "spokeswoman" rather than "spokesperson".

Check with the organisation for the term they use; if in doubt, use "chairman".

Use the plural to avoid clumsy constructions (for example, write "Doctors prescribe the best drugs for their patients.", not "A doctor prescribes the best drug for his or her patients."). Avoid any form of sexist language.

Words often interchanged

As a rule of thumb, always use the shorter and clearer alternative if you have one or more alternatives to choose from.

A or an

The use of "a" or "an" depends on the sound at the start of the following word, i.e. it does not depend on the way we write the following word, it depends on the way we say it.

If the following word starts with a consonant sound, then we say a (for example, "a patient", "a treatment", "a side effect"), whereas if the following word starts with a vowel sound, then we say an (for example, "an interesting case", "an extremely complicated operation", "an adverse event").

Normally, consonant letters are pronounced with a consonant sound, and vowel letters with a vowel sound. However, there are some exceptions, for instance in abbreviations, even though the rule about **a** or **an** is the same.

Remember to think about the sound, not the writing. Therefore, vowel letters with consonant sounds indicate a (for example, "a once-daily treatment", "a European guideline", a "University degree"), and consonant letters with vowel sounds (for example, "an honest answer", "an hour", "an SMS text", "an FDA guideline") indicate an.

Administer or provide or give

An administrator administers various affairs in an administration. Although it is accepted throughout the literature to administer medicine, use the shorter alternative, i.e. give (for example, "The doctor provided or gave ibuprofen for pain relief", instead of "the doctor administered ibuprofen for pain relief.").

Adopt or use

The word "use" is less likely to be misunderstood by the reader (for example, "The doctor chose to use the invasive procedure", instead of "the doctor chose to adopt the invasive procedure.").

Adverse events or adverse reactions:

An "adverse event" is a medical occurrence temporally associated with the use of a drug, but not necessarily causally related.

An "adverse reaction" is a response to a drug which is noxious and unintended, and which occurs at doses normally used in man for the prophylaxis, diagnosis, or therapy of disease, or for the modifications of physiological function. Adverse events and reactions can be serious or non-serious.

Advocate or suggest

Advocate means to defend, plead, act or speak on behalf of another person or group of people. Do not use advocate if you wish to communicate that something has been suggested (for example, "the investigators suggested the new drug was more effective that the comparator", rather than "the investigators advocated the new drug was more effective that the comparator").

Aetiology or cause

Cause means the cause itself, which is what an author is usually trying to communicate, rather than the aetiology, which means the study of the causes of diseases. Therefore, unless you are talking about the science of the causes, use cause (for example, "we investigated the cause of inflammation", rather than "we studied the aetiology of inflammation").

Amount or quantity or number

The word "amount" is a characteristic, as of energy or mass, susceptible of precise physical measurement (for example, "the doctor undertook an inordinate amount of work").

The term "quantity" is used for things that you can measure (for example, "the Director took control of a large quantity of money"), whereas "number of" precedes a plural, a countable noun (for example, "the disease affected a large number of patients").

Data or results

"Data" is the background information that enables the analysis leading to "results". For example, "the trial data has been collected and will now be analysed", and "once the data is analysed we will have the results".

Demonstrate or show

To "demonstrate" something is to clearly and deliberately manifest something (for example, "the young doctor clearly demonstrated her surgical skills"). To show something is less specific (for example, "the boy showed the doctor where it hurt").

Efficacy or effectiveness

The words efficacy and effectiveness are interchangeable in most situations. Both words are defined as measuring something to determine the ability to produce an effect.

In science and medicine, the word efficacy is preferred when describing the effectiveness of a particular treatment or drug (for example, "the efficacy of the drug was assessed during the study".

The word effective, however, is not limited to describing medical situations (for example, "the effectiveness of the treatment is questionable").

Elevate or increase

Elevate means to raise something up to a higher level, position, or state (for example, "the head of the patient was elevated by a pillow", whereas increase means become greater or larger (for example, "the number of emergency visits increased during 2012").

Encounter or find

An encounter is something that is unexpected or unplanned (for example, "the doctor encountered an old patient in the cafeteria"), whereas found means to reach, recover or acquire something (for example, "the nurse found the scalpel before closing the wound").

Explore or study

To explore is to systematically investigate or examine something (for example, "the doctors have explored every treatment option"). Study is the pursuit of knowledge or increasing knowledge by reading, observing or through research (for example, "the student needed to study to pass the exam").

Following or after

To follow means coming next in time or order (for example, "I will see the following patients before lunch"), whereas after refers to behind in place or order, and next to or lower than in order or importance (for example, "I will see the remaining patients after lunch").

Here and our

Do not assume that "here" means the same to the reader as it does to the author (for example, here to someone in Copenhagen does not mean the same as here to someone in London).

Do not assume the audience has the same attitude as the author, as this could cause offence (for example, write "the hospital's view on the treatment is…", not "our views on the treatment is…").

Hypothesis or guess

A hypothesis is an educated guess, while a guess has no previous knowledge about the subject.

A hypothesis is usually part of a scientific experiment which involves a statistical method for testing the hypothesis, and either supporting it, or supporting the opposite (the so called null hypothesis).

A hypothesis is a guess made after research has been done, while a guess is made without previous knowledge of the question, before any research.

Effect or affect or impact

The main difference between "affect" and "effect" is that in most cases affect is used as a verb, whereas, effect is used as a noun. Affect means to have an influence on something (for example, "the drug affected the healing process".

However, affect as a noun has a specialised meaning in medicine and psychology, referring to moods and feeling as distinct from thoughts or knowledge.

Effect, on the other hand, denotes a result, i.e. it is a consequence (for example, "the medicine had a healing effect"). Impact, however, is physical contact such as a punch in the face, or being hit by a car.

The word "impact" as a verb means strike with a blow or to pack firmly together (for example, "due to arthritis the femur impacted the tibia"). Impact as a noun means a collision, punch etc. (for example, "the impact of the crash resulted in multiple injuries to the driver").

Do not use impact as a verb in place of affect (for example "the temperature impacts the growth rate of bacteria". Instead write "the temperature affects the growth rate of bacteria").

Do not use impact as a noun in place of effect (for example, "refined carbohydrates have significant impact on the increased prevalence of childhood obesity". Instead write "refined carbohydrates have significant effect on the increased prevalence of childhood obesity").

Elusive or illusive

The word "elusive" means hard to find, catch, or achieve (for example, "the new operation proved elusive to perform"), whereas "illusive" means not real although appearing so (for example, "the doctor tried to understand the illusive mind of the psychotic patient").

I, me or myself

The word "myself" is a reflective noun which is basically a word that expresses something you do to yourself (for example, "I love myself", "I thought to myself I'm hungry", "bought myself a bottle of wine").

Notice that the word myself is always paired with the word "I". Myself can also be an intensive pronoun, meaning you would like to emphasise that you, in fact, did something (for example, "I myself performed the operation and saved the patient's life").

The word I goes before the verb (for example, "I went to the clinic"). The word "me" goes after the verb (for example, "the doctor gave the medicine to me"). If you are in doubt, use I or me.

It

Do not confuse the reader when you use this pronoun. Never sacrifice clarity (for example, "she connected the machine to the rabbit and it exploded".

This means the rabbit exploded – which is probably not what you are attempting to communicate. Instead, be clear and write "she connected the machine to the rabbit and the machine exploded.").

Language

Use a short, simple word rather than a longer word (long words make sentences more difficult to read). However, do not sacrifice clarity for brevity. Avoid using unnecessary foreign or Latin phrases (for example, sine qua non, persona non grata, de rigueur, en passant, per capita).

Consider replacing the following long(er) words with shorter ones. As a rule of thumb with "as" (in the sense of "in the way that" or "in the same way"), "as if" or "as though", then "like" is incorrect (for example, write "He treats that patient like a baby", not "He treats that patient like a mother treats a baby.").

Less or fewer

"Fewer" is used if you are referring to people or things in the plural (e.g. hospitals, books, patients, students, children). Use "less" when you are referring to something that cannot be counted or does not have a plural (e.g. money, air, time, rain). See more about less and fewer under volume and quantity.

Location or place

The location of an area provides a reference to locate a place. A location can be absolute or relative. Absolute location provides a definite reference to the area (for example, latitude and longitude, city or town name, or a street address).

Relative location describes the area with respect to its environment and its connection to other places. A place, on the other hand, generally describes the characteristics of the location (for example, beaches, mountains and rivers).

May or might

May or might, both are the way of expressing possibility. May is to have the permission (for example, "the patient may go home"), and might is to make a possibility less likely (for example, "the experiment might cure the patient").

Money

Use the numeric form for sums less than one million (for example, "57 500 GBP for research").

Use the mixed (number and character) form for sums greater than one million (for example, "a total budget of 5 million GBP").

Always indicate the currency (for example, "37.50 USD" for American dollars, "37.50 CAD" for Canadian dollars, "37.50 GBP" for British pounds).

Following the number, write an appropriate abbreviation for other well-known currencies (for example, "37.50 DKK" for Danish kroner).

Following the number, write the full name of the currency for lesser-known currencies (for example, "37 Haitian gourds").

Monitor or measure

Monitor refers to keeping track of something systematically by collecting information, i.e. the actual data recovery and collection process, whereas when you measure the dimensions, quantity, or capacity as ascertained by comparison with a standard, i.e. evaluating the process with the final outcome.

Morphology or shape

Morphology is the study of the form (shape) and structure of organisms without consideration of function, whereas shape refers to the configuration of an object, i.e. its outline or contour.

Novel or new

Novel means a new kind, i.e. different from anything seen or known before (for example, "Einstein's theory of relativity was novel", while new refers to recent origin, production, purchase, etc. having lately come or been brought into being (for example, "I have a new textbook in my collection").

Only or just

Avoid using the words "only" and "just" unless you mean to infer an opinion (instead write, for example, "less than").

Optimum/optimal or best

Optimum means most favourable or most conducive to a given end especially under fixed conditions whereas optimal refers to something that is most desirable or satisfactory. Best is a superlative that compares more than two items or processes (good, better and best). If two items are compared, one is "better" than the other.

Pathology or disease

Pathology is the science of the causes and effects of a disease, whereas a disease is a disorder of structure or function in a living organism.

Patient or subject

Clinical pharmacology studies generally include subjects (for example, "healthy subjects", "subjects with renal impairment"). Phase 2 and 3 studies include patients.

If a protocol has not used these terms as above, then use as in the protocol. Use the disease as something the patients have rather than in the adjectival form (for example, write "patients with diabetes" not "diabetic patients").

People and animals

People less than 18 years of age are "boys" and "girls". "Adolescents" can be used if the age range is defined. People more than 18 years of age are "men" and "women".

Do not use the words "youths" or "ladies". Animals are "male" and "female" (for example, "female Rhesus monkeys").

Per

In statistical or technical contexts, per is acceptable if it means "for each" (for example, "Sixty-six per cent of patients reached full remission."). For exposure, write "per 100 patient-years of exposure". Write "a year", not "per annum". Write "a person" or "each", not "per person". Write "hourly", not "per hour". Write "daily", not "per day".

Possess or have

Possess means to own or to have as a quality (for example, "the bullet is safe in the doctor's possession"). It is also used in other situations (for example, "what possessed the patient to take an overdose?").

Have is to approach possession (for example, "can I have a glass of water?").

Prior to or before

Although prior to is used extensively in medical texts, the meaning of prior to and before is the same. Therefore, as a rule of thumb, use the simpler and shorter before.

Race

If you mention race, use the descriptions that people use of themselves (for example, in the United Kingdom, people of African origin are usually "Black" and people from the Indian subcontinent are often "Asian").

In the United States, people of African origin are "African American" (this might, however, become confusing if you are talking about people from e.g. Jamaica).

Where possible, be more specific. In clinical study reports, unless specified otherwise, use "Black", "Caucasian", "Asian", and "Other".

Rationale or reason

The rationale is the argument for something while the reason is the purpose, so the two can be quite different (for example, "the rationale for the surgery was the patient had a tumour, but the reason was to remove the tumour".

Reveal or show

To reveal is to make something unknown known (for example, "the doctor revealed the new results at the conference") whereas to show is to bring something to view whether it is known or unknown (for example, "a week after her hip surgery she wanted to show the doctor that she could walk").

Sample or group

In statistics, a sample is a set of elements drawn from and analysed to estimate the characteristics of a population (for example, "the trial investigated a sample of the population").

A sample can also be a portion or a piece (for example, "the doctor took a sample of the tumour").

A group is an assemblage of people, animals or other objects gathered or located together (for example, "the doctor invited a group of people to celebrate his birthday").

Speciality and specialty

Specialities are distinguishing marks or features (for instance, "the pizza is an Italian speciality"), whereas cardiology, neurology psychiatry etc. are specialties. In the USA specialty is used for both meanings.

Superior or better

Superior means above (for example, "the head is located superior to the neck"), while better describes a comparison of quality, improvement etc. (for example, "the new drug works better than the old one").

Visualise or see

Visualise is relating to the sense of sight, projections and images through optic instruments x-rays etc. (for example, "the structure was only visual through the microscope").

See or seen means to perceive with the eye, and is almost always a better word to use instead of visualise (for example "The doctor wanted to see the tumour").

Geography

Use the English spelling of place names (for example, write "Vienna" not "Wien"). Remember, Holland is not The Netherlands and that Scandinavia is not a synonym for the Nordic countries.

Be accurate, precise, and without prejudice.

Said

The simple, unequivocal "said" is always preferred in attribution. Words like "admitted", "agreed", "concluded", "continued", and "commented" all have shades of meaning that interfere with objectivity in reporting.

Use words other than "said" only in exceptional circumstances. Use the

form: "The new MS drug has changed my life, the patient said." Not "…
said the patient."

Study and patient ID

For specified studies, use uppercase "S" and do not use "No."; use a non-
breaking space (for example, write "Study PH-201", "Studies PH-001 and
PH-003"). For specified patients, use uppercase "P" and do not use "No.";
use a non-breaking space (for example, "Patient 1234", "Patients 1234 and
5678").

Study or trial

"Study" is the preferred term. Use "trial" if it is part of a specific term (for
example, "Trial Master File").

Tautology

Do not say the same thing twice using different words (for example, "repeat
again", "new innovation", "different alternative", "general consensus",
"close proximity", "future prospects", "full potential", "past history",
"essential prerequisite", "8:30 pm at night", "2 am in the morning", "actual
facts", "the reason why", "the reason … is because …".

Do not use "earlier" or "later" if it says the same thing more than once in
different ways without adding clarity (for example, "A speech given earlier
today …" reports a speech before the text was written, so "earlier" should
be deleted).

Time

Write the time of day in text in formal writing (for example, "Give the dose
at six o'clock in the morning."). Use numbers to emphasise an exact time,
and use a non-breaking space (for example, "The dose was received at
18:35").

Always write numbers when "am" or "pm" is used (for example, 7:00 am or
6:35 pm). Some specific clinical studies may require more specific times (for
example, "16:09:41.3"). Write "next week", "last month", or "on
Wednesday" and include the actual date in brackets as confirmation.

Versus

This Latin preposition should be italicised (for example, "Ibuprofen versus placebo"). Never use it as a verb (for example, do not write "Ibuprofen will versus placebo"). Use the abbreviation in tables (for example, "ESC vs. PBO")

Names and titles

Trade names

Unless necessary, use the generic name for medications. Generic names are never capitalised. Trade names must be recognised and the capital retained (for example, "Polaroid", "Xerox"), or there can be legal repercussions from the owners of the trade names.

Some trade names no longer carry the capital (for example, thermos, nylon, pyrex, cellophane). If in doubt, use the generic name (for example, write "instant photograph" not "Polaroid").

Trademarks

Use caution when writing about patents or trademarks. If you are in any doubt about what to write, contact the source.

As an author for a company you are obligated to use the trademark or registered-trademark symbol (™ or ®, not a footnote) after the product names.

This also applies to products that are not owned by the company you are writing for. Use the trademark or registered trademark symbol (™ or ®) no more than three times in one article for each trade name. For example:

- the first mention in the article's title
- the first mention in the abstract or synopsis
- the first mention in the article's text

If the article is part of a symposium, add symbols to the trade names in question in all other articles in the symposium for consistency. In general, treat corporation names as trade names – spell them as the corporation spells them.

Personal names

At first mention, give a person's full name without title (for example, "Jenny Smith"). However, if the title is relevant (such as a professional title), include it (for example, "Professor Pauline Pope"); at subsequent mentions, use the title and the surname (for example, "Ms Smith", "Professor Pope"). Use the English order of names.

In some languages, a diminutive name may be used instead of the formal name (for example, diminutive name for Frederik is Fred, Bradley is Brad and William is Will). Do not use spaces or full stops with initials (for example, "PD James").

Personal names with "Jr" (Junior) or "Sr" (Senior)

Use a comma between the name and "Jr" or "Sr" (for example, "William Johns, Jr"). Use a comma between these abbreviations and any degrees or titles that follow (for example, "William Johns, Jr, MD"). Do not use a comma to separate a name from the titles "II," "III," or "IV" (for example, "Charles Forsythe III")

Titles and ranks

Use Mr, Ms, Mrs, Dr, Professor, Associate Professor, Sir (only Mr, Ms, Dr, and Mrs should be used as contractions). At second and subsequent references, "Professor" and "Associate Professor" are both written as "Professor" (not "Prof." or "Assoc. Prof.").

Do not use professions as titles when they are not (for example, write "John Johnson, physiotherapist" or "physiotherapist, John Johnson"; not "physiotherapist John Johnson").

Chiropractor is not a title, so "Mark Smith, chiropractor", becomes "Dr Smith" next time he is mentioned.

With the exception of those titles listed under Abbreviations, titles are given in full, along with the person's full name, at the first mention of a person. They are abbreviated only at subsequent mentions.

Academic qualifications

Do not use full stops in abbreviations for academic qualifications (for example, BSc, MSc, MD, PhD). Use lowercase and an apostrophe in "bachelor's degree" and "master's degree" (for example, "a bachelor's degree in biochemistry").

Do not use a courtesy title when an abbreviation follows the name (for example, write "John Jones, PhD" or "Dr John Jones"; not "Dr John Jones, PhD").

For physicians, use their academic title first and refer to them as "Dr" after that (for example, "Jack Barnes, MD, chaired the debate … Dr Barnes' views on this subject are well known.").

Addresses

For numbered addresses, use abbreviations such as Ave, Blvd, Rd, St (for example, "134 Oxford St" and "4316 Sunset Blvd"). For unnumbered addresses, write out and capitalise the street name (for example, "Sunset Boulevard").

4 UNITS, NAMES AND MEASUREMENTS

General info

In general, numbers from zero to ten are spelled out, and numbers 11 and higher are written as numerals. However, exceptions occur more frequently than not.

One exception is that we should not mix numerals with the spelled out versions within the same list or context (for example, do not write: "At the birthday party, one child cried, and 11 children had great fun.").

Units of measurement

Always use numerals with units when the context is statistical. This includes the following:

- Units of measurement: 56 cm, 5 mmol, 0.4 kg
- Time: 5 hours, 7 days' treatment, 18-week study, 2 years old
- Subjects or patients in a study: 300 subjects were randomised, 3 patients died
- AEs, SAEs, TEAEs: There were 4 AE withdrawals.
- Studies or trials: …across the 5 trials…
- Fold: 3-fold, 10-fold, 25-fold.

Intervals and ranges of numbers

Ranges of numbers always take the en-dash: 300–350 patients, 25–30 g. Check for proper syntax when using numbers.

If you write from, you must also write to. If you write between, you must also write and:

- "Between 50 and 100 subjects", not "Between 50–100 subjects"
- "Means ranged from 4.6 to 5.6", not "Means ranged from 4.6–5.6"
- Mean range was 4.6–5.6.

Units of time

When talking about spans of time that are actually data points, always use numerals (for example, "women should be post-menopausal for at least 1 year before participating in the trial. Patients were dosed for 6 weeks."). Note also the following acceptable formats:

- 6 weeks of treatment

- 6 weeks' treatment

- 6-week treatment.

Decimals, fractions and precision

When discussing numbers less than 1, always use the plural:

- 0 hours

- 0.5 days

- meters but 1 meter

- 1/8 inches or one-eighth of an inch.

Try to be consistent with respect to precision (for example, "doses were either 1 or 1.5 mL" should be changed to "doses were either 1.0 or 1.5 mL").

Bullet list

Bullet text is for the brief line of introduction before the bullets begin. No extra line space appears after it, and it will be kept together with the list, never separated by a page break.

Typing Return after bullet text will automatically give you the first bullet. Bullet list and bullet list numbered provide standard formatting for bulleted and numbered lists. Indents provide formatting for sub-lists inside a bulleted or numbered list, giving an automatic indent, and – instead of bullets.

End punctuation with bulleted lists

If a bullet point is a complete sentence, it should end with a full stop. Incomplete sentences should not. Non-sentences used together with complete sentences, however, may both take a full stop, as shown below.

It is acceptable for a bullet list to have a mixture of points ending with and without full stops. For example, "Patients are to be treated as follows:

- Fairly
- With compassion
- They must receive their prescribed doses according to the dosing schedule.
- In order. Investigators must refer to the alphabetised list.
- Some patients were excluded. Excluded patients were later rescreened.

Numbers

Use zero followed by a decimal point for numbers less than one (for example, 0.5). Use text and hyphens for fractions (for example, write "one-third of the patients were men" not "1/3 of patients were men").

Use numbers with decimal points (for example, write "37.8°C" not "thirty-seven point eight"). Write 1000 not 1,000. Write 10 000 not 10,000 (except for page numbers).

Use text for ordinal numbers less than 100 (for example, write "second", "eleventh", "twenty-second"). Use 'to' in an interval rather than a hyphen (for example, write "aged 18 to 65 years" not "aged 18-65 years").

Use figures for counted numbers and measurements (for example, "3 patients"). Use text for items that are not counted or measured (for example, "two treatment groups"). Avoid starting a sentence with numbers, unless very simple (for example, One, Two, One million).

If numbers are used to start a sentence, use text (for example, "Sixty-three of the patients treated with this antidepressant were complete remitters.", but the preferred format is "A total of 63 patients treated . . .").

Do not write numbers as text and then repeat as figures in parentheses (for example, do not write "Five (5) . . ."). In telephone numbers, do not use hyphens (for example, write "020 1234 1234" not "020-1234-1234").

The country code should be preceded using "+", and parentheses should be used to separate the country code and city or regional codes from the local phone number (for example, "+44 (0)20 1234 1234"). Telephone numbers may be used in protocols, but never in clinical study reports.

When rounding numbers, if the final digit is 1 to 4, round down (for example, round 2.24 down to 2.2) and round up when the digit is 6 to 9, (for example, round 2.26 up to 2.3).

When rounding numbers, if the final digit is 5 and the preceding digit is even, round down (for example, round 2.245 down to 2.24) and round up when it is odd (for example, round 2.255 up to 2.26).

When rounding numbers, keep in mind that a number that ends in "5" may itself be a rounded figure (always check the original data).

Be careful when using "a factor of" and "increase of 23%" to describe changes or differences. If the unit of measurement is "%", use "increase of xx percentage points".

Use a non-breaking space between "Figure" and the number (for example, "Figure 1").

Write the following statistical terms as:

- "P" for P values (for example, P = 0.05 and P >0.05). Use a non-breaking space after "P" and after "="
- "degrees of freedom" (df) (written out)
- "SEM" ("standard error of the mean") and "SD" ("standard deviation")
- "χ^2-test" (Greek letter chi [χ] followed by superscript "2")
- T-test
- CI ("confidence interval").

Space around numbers and operators

As a rule, always put space between a number and its unit (for example, "5 mL", "12 hours", "500 g"). Exceptions are for example, "100%", "25°C".

Operators such as ~, <, >, ≤, ≥, ×, +, – and ± are sometimes are used with space, sometimes not. The difference is grammatical. For example, < can mean less than, and it can also mean is less than.

In the first case, the symbol is an adjective. In the second case, it is a verb.

When the symbol is being used as an adjective, do not use space (for example, "He had a BMI of >29.9", "The SD was ±0.5 mm.", "Growth rate was 2× the mean", "For ~24 hours.").

When the symbol is used as a verb, as often the case in equations, there must be space on both sides of the symbol (for example, "Subjects with BMI ≥ 29.9" (open), but "Subjects with a BMI of ≥29.9" (closed), and "P < 0.001".

Note the equals sign (=) always has space on both sides (for example, "NPG = nocturnal plasma glucose", and "x + y = z". Note also, the solidus (/) never uses space but is always closed on both sides (for example, "6/7", "x/y", "benefit/risk").

Measurements

Use a non-breaking space in Word between the number and the units of measure (for example, use "4 L [with a non-breaking space]", not "4L" nor "4 L [ordinary space]" for "four litres"). If you want to insert a non-breaking space, press CTRL+SHIFT+SPACEBAR (Microsoft Word).

Examples of exceptions, write "37.8°C", not "37.8 °C" or "37.8 ° C", and if you do not have the """ symbol available, you can write "37.8 degrees Celsius". Write 37%, not 37 %.

Write "six-foot man" and "six feet, three inches". Write "Ten milligrams was given daily.", not "Ten milligrams were given daily.".

Use only one solidus (/) in each expression (for example, write "6 mL/mg per minute" not "6 mL/mg/minute").

Tables

Use a non-breaking space between "Table" and the number (for example, "Table 1"). Do not use "see" in running text, refer to each table using an

Arabic numeral (for example, write "50% remitters (Table 1)", not "50% remitters, see Table 1").

5 USING ABBREVIATIONS AND ACRONYMS

An abbreviation's sole function is to aid the reader, not the writer. Without abbreviations, the reader might have to wade through heavy, repetitious text, without any added understanding.

However, too many abbreviations and a document starts to lose its ability to provide a coherent meaning.

Keep the reader in mind when using abbreviations. If an abbreviation is used three times or fewer, just spell it out, and delete the term from the list of abbreviations.

An exception to this could be invoked if two or more occurrences all appear in the same paragraph or on the same page.

Abbreviations may be defined more than once in the same document to help the reader, especially if there have been many pages or sections since the abbreviation's last use, or if the abbreviation is not very common or familiar.

Abbreviation consistency

If an abbreviation is defined in the list of abbreviations, but not used in the main text or appendices, it should be deleted from the list of abbreviations.

Note: Some abbreviations are not used in text, but are used in tables or figures. For those, the abbreviations should be defined in the footnote of each table or figure in which it appears (tables and figures should always be able to stand alone).

Table and figure abbreviations do not need to be defined in the list of abbreviations, but to do so might be helpful.

If an abbreviation is used only rarely in a document, check to see if it will be used in appendix documents (for example, with protocols or IBs) before deleting it from the list of abbreviations. The list of abbreviations is meant to cover the text part as well as all appended documents.

Acronyms

Acronyms are formed from the first letters of groups of words. Some acronyms have become words (for example, "laser") and others are pronounced as words (for example, FDA or EMA).

Most should be written in full at first reference, followed by the acronym in brackets (for example, "World Health Organisation (WHO)").

Plural of abbreviations and acronyms

Use the singular for most common abbreviations, even when they refer to more than one item (for example, write "p 5 to 6" for "pages 5 to 6" in references).

In text, always write "pages 5 to 6", never "p 5 to 6". Plurals of abbreviations and acronyms are formed by adding an "s", without an apostrophe (for example, "MDs").

6 ETHICAL CONSIDERATIONS IN MEDICAL COMMUNICATION

The pharmaceutical industry provides a valid and legitimate contribution to society. At the same time, the pharmaceutical industry is a business heavily dependent on marketing. The greater the volume of products sold, the greater the return of investment.

When product sales are given priority over public health, promotion can lead to over-prescribing as well as poor quality prescribing and medicine use. This, in turn, leads to an increased risk of adverse events and higher healthcare costs.

Prescribers often find themselves trapped between patients' needs and healthcare priorities on one hand, and promotional influences on the other.

Dual allegiances and conflicts of interest can cloud judgement and cause distortions in both the delivery of healthcare and the conduct of research in medicine.

Physicians, pharmacists, researchers, educators, managers and administrators need practical guidance on how to implement its marketing practices so that health outcomes are enhanced.

The World Medical Association states that the key ethical basis for any guidance is the understanding that the values of clinical care, of welfare of society and of science should prevail over commercial imperatives and monetary concerns.

Scandals leading to improved ethics

A number of scandals involving unethical use of various products have led to strict laws and regulations about the communication associated with marketed products as well as drugs and devices in development.

One well-known example is the thalidomide scandal in the late 1950s and early 1960s, which left a lasting global effect.

Thalidomide was released as a sedative drug in 1957, and it was also found to ease the effects of morning sickness in pregnant women. In 1962 thalidomide was withdrawn from the market after it was discovered that it interfered with developing foetuses and caused severe birth defects.

At that time, scientists did not even think that drugs taken by a pregnant woman could harm the foetus. Ultimately, thousands of pregnant women took thalidomide during its five years on the market and over 10 000 children were born with defects.

Many other cruel and painful experiments have been carried out throughout the history of medical research. This has led to several initiatives, e.g. the Nuremberg Code and the Helsinki Declaration, where ethical principles regarding human research were developed to safeguard each individual taking part in both medical research and treatment.

Ethics is the application of a moral code to the practice of science and medicine. What and how you communicate to ethics committees is crucial for a successful outcome. The law demands that patients are treated the way you would wish to be treated yourself.

Ethics in medicine has advanced to an extent that healthcare professionals are likely to be faced with controversial issues on a regular basis.

For example, euthanasia (intentionally ending a life in order to relieve pain and suffering), collection and use of human tissue and information sharing are typical where clinicians must be up to date on the current legislation and thus ensure that they follow it.

This chapter gives an overview of the most important points in medical ethics.

Caring for each patient as an individual

Providing each patient with the best possible individual treatment and caring for them with dignity and respect are important principles. Efficient use of resources often makes the care of patients difficult.

As a consequence, the interests of economic restraints and legal boundaries must also be considered in the treatment of each patient.

Patients should be provided with the best possible care irrespective of prejudicing factors such as age, sexuality, ethnicity, religious beliefs or politics.

The same goes for a number of lifestyle issues like smoking, obesity and alcohol or drug abuse. The healthcare provider has a duty to always be supportive, not judgmental.

Good clinical practice

As part of doing the best for patients, healthcare providers must also maintain a good standard of clinical practice. Medicine is rapidly evolving and it is a fundamental requirement that both knowledge and skills are kept up-to-date.

Healthcare providers must always (wherever possible) practise evidence-based medicine. Good clinical practice also means always being thorough and ensuring that sufficient time is devoted to provide safe and effective care for each patient.

Confidentiality

Strict confidentiality must be kept at all times. Breach of confidentiality may have serious consequences for both the patient and the healthcare provider.

In rare occasions, the obligations to the safety of others and the greater public good must override the duty of confidentiality to a patient, such as the disclosure of serious communicable diseases and reporting of serious crimes etc.

Informed consent

It is not enough simply to obtain consent from a patient. The consent must be informed. It is important that a sufficient amount of information is provided and that it is presented in a way that the patient understands.

Informed consent not only applies to procedures or operations, but also to all medical interventions, including the prescribing of medicinal products.

Potential risks and side effects should be presented for the patient, but it is always difficult to decide what to include and what to omit, since every single treatment is more or less associated with a certain risk.

A very low risk can be omitted but it may become more important if it results in a side effect that turns out to be serious or fatal. Communicating risks are useless if the patient does not understand them. To make the message as clear as possible, try to avoid jargon, technical terms and abbreviations that may create confusion for the patient.

When communicating about the patient with family, relatives and friends, the default position is to obtain each patient's consent. Written consent is always best, but if it is verbal it must still be properly documented in the patient records.

Furthermore, if someone other than the patient raises any concerns with healthcare providers, no guarantees should be given that the discussion will be kept from the patient.

Where a patient lacks the capacity to make an informed decision about whether information should be disclosed or not the healthcare provider must make the patients interest's the primary concern by protecting patient privacy, integrity and best interests.

In such situations the healthcare provider may need to share information with individuals authorised to represent the patient, but this does not mean allowing free access to all information.

Consent in minors

When obtaining consent from a child, the healthcare provider needs to establish whether the child is legally competent to give consent. People aged 16 and over are legally presumed to have the capacity to consent to treatment unless there is evidence to the contrary.

If a child is deemed not legally competent, consent needs to be obtained from a parent or someone with parental responsibility. However, this does not apply in emergencies, where treatment can be provided without consent to save the life, or prevent serious deterioration of health, of the patient.

Aspects to look out for

Ethics is mostly common sense but there may be different opinions and more than one correct answer.

Make sure that you record ethical considerations in the patient charts along with other medical decisions. Always ensure the welfare of your patient by being open and honest.

Patients have the right to make bad decisions but no matter what, you need to provide relevant and correct information. You cannot force patients to choose healthy lifestyles.

Sane people are also permitted to refuse effective, even life-saving treatment. Not everyone may share your views and values and they have a right to disagree.

You have a right to express your views but not to enforce them, but you should be prepared to justify your position.

7 WRITING FOR MARKETING AND ADVERTISING

Writing advertisements for professionals

Although national legislations differ considerably between countries, the law requires specific information to be provided when you are communicating to healthcare professionals.

Such information includes the product's name, a list of active ingredients using the generic name presented in connection with the product name, the classification for the sale or supply of the product, one or more of the product's indications and the route or method of administration, if it is not obvious.

A clear and legible summarised statement of the information from the approved summary of product characteristics (SmPC) regarding adverse reactions, special precautions and important contraindications, dosage and method of use relevant to the specific indications must be presented within the advertisement to enable the reader to easily understand the relationship between this information and the claims as well as indications of the product.

The name and address of the marketing authorisation holder, and the address of the part of the business responsible for placing the medicinal product on the market, as well as certification of registration or certificate of traditional use registration, should also be provided along with the authorisation number.

If applicable, the words "traditional herbal medicinal product for use in", followed by one or more therapeutic-approved indications, and followed by the words "exclusively based upon long-standing use", should be included.

Separate requirements exist for abbreviated reminder advertisements. The pharmaceutical code adds that this information should be clear, legible and an integral part of the promotional material.

Writing advertisements for patients

Advertising of non-prescription, over the counter (OTC), medicines to the general public is permitted based on the requirements of the specific national regulations.

Before a medicinal product can be advertised, it must be the subject of a marketing authorisation (MA) or a certification of traditional use (in respect of herbal medicinal products).

Everything advertised prior to the MA is considered as pre-launch communication, which is not allowed.

The advertisement must be accurate, to the point and fairly present the claim of the product objectively, and be totally consistent with the terms provided with the MA and the SmPC of the product, and encourage rational use of the product.

The information may not contain material which:

- provides the impression that a medical consultation or surgical operation is unnecessary and can be substituted by offering treatment or diagnosis in other ways, e.g. through a website
- provides the impression that the effects of the medicinal product are guaranteed, adverse events/reactions are clearly listed, are better/superior, more effective than, or equivalent to, those of another treatment or product
- provides the impression that the product promotes or improves health, or is necessary for the health of the patient or that the health of the patient could be deteriorated by not taking the product
- provides the impression that the product possesses a special effect or quality which is unknown, unrecognised or unpublished
- is intended exclusively for children, or might result in any harm to children or exploit their innocence and inexperience to objectively and critically evaluate the information
- is endorsed by any credible person or organisation suggesting that the product is a food, cosmetics or other consumer products
- provides the impression that the safety or efficacy of the product is due to the fact that it is natural
- provides an impression that may lead to erroneous self-diagnosis

- provides improper, alarming or misleading terms to claims of recovery.

The law includes requirements about the form and content of advertisements where the product must be clearly identified as a medicinal product, and it must include a certain minimum of information, e.g. the name of the product and instructions for use.

The law also includes requirements stating that advertisements must be accurate, truthful and easily intelligible for the intended audience. Furthermore it:

- should not bring the industry into disrepute
- should not offer treatment for a serious disease requiring intervention by a healthcare professional
- should not offer to treat by correspondence
- should not exaggerate or influence consumers, or refer to specialists or tests, unless it can be scientifically substantiated.

Although the rules differ between countries, a number of OTC products should not be promoted to the general public, including various analgesics and antihistamines. The law also prohibits exaggerated claims in advertising, as well as making disparaging references to other producer's products, services or promotions.

The use of competitor's brands or logos is not permitted unless appropriate consent has been received. Comparisons with rival products must be factual, fair and capable of substantiation.

In most countries it is also prohibited to advertise a product as being new if it has been available on the market for more than 12 months. It is generally also prohibited to use the word "safe" or "effective" in an advertisement without qualification.

8 COMMUNICATING RESEARCH

Different types of research are presented in various ways. There are many types of studies that are designed to answer specific questions.

In pharmaceutical development, a variety of different topics related to quality, safety and efficacy are studied throughout the development phases.

In total, the average new drug takes about 10 - 15 years to develop from discovery to approval for marketing. Bringing a new drug to market involves a series of research stages and regulatory approvals. The different processes and phases are:

Discovery

The work at this stage is mostly conducted in a laboratory and may take several years to yield results. It involves identifying molecules or processes responsible for a particular application, then searching for compounds that might act against those targets.

Once a potential compound is found, it is modified many times over to improve its drug properties.

Tests are done in cellular and animal models to learn more about the compound's mechanisms of action against a particular application. If these experiments are successful, the compound moves into pre-clinical testing.

The pre-clinical, or non-clinical, research and development

This is where a potential drug is tested for its safety and efficacy (effectiveness) in an appropriate animal model.

The results from pre-clinical research determine whether there is sufficient potential for a drug to proceed to testing in human clinical trials. Pre-clinical testing commonly takes one to three years to complete.

Clinical research and development

Phase 1

Phase 1 studies assess the safety of a drug or device. This initial phase of testing, which can take several months to complete, usually includes a small number of healthy volunteers (20 to 100), who are generally paid for participating in the study.

The study is designed to determine the effects of the drug or device on humans including how it is absorbed, metabolised, and excreted. This phase also investigates the side effects that occur as dosage levels are increased. About 70% of experimental drugs pass this phase of testing.

Phase 2

Phase 2 studies test the efficacy of a drug or device. This second phase of testing can last from several months to two years, and involves up to several hundred patients.

Most phase 2 studies are randomised trials where one group of patients receives the experimental drug, while a second "control" group receives a standard treatment or placebo.

Often these studies are "blinded" which means that neither the patients nor the researchers know who has received the experimental drug.

This allows investigators to provide the pharmaceutical company and the health authorities with comparative information about the relative safety and effectiveness of the new drug. About one-third of experimental drugs successfully complete both phase 1 and phase 2 studies.

Phase 3

Phase 3 studies involve randomised and blind testing in several hundred to several thousand patients.

This large-scale testing, which can last several years, provides the pharmaceutical company and the health authorities with a more thorough understanding of the effectiveness of the drug or device, the benefits and the range of possible adverse reactions. 70% to 90% of drugs that enter phase 3 studies successfully complete this phase of testing. Once phase 3 is complete, a pharmaceutical company can request the authorities for approval to market the product.

Postmarketing

Phase 4

Phase 4 studies, often called post marketing surveillance trials, are conducted after a drug or device has been approved for consumer use.

Pharmaceutical companies have several objectives at this stage: (1) to compare a drug with other drugs already on the market, (2) to monitor a drug's long-term effectiveness and impact on a patient's quality of life, and (3) to determine the cost-effectiveness of a drug therapy relative to other traditional and new therapies.

Phase 4 studies can result in a drug or device being taken off the market or restrictions of use could be placed on the product depending on the findings in the study.

Study types

Observational studies

Here researchers observe the effect of a risk factor, diagnostic test or treatment without trying to influence what happens.

Such studies are usually "retrospective", i.e. the data are based on events that have already happened. Most workplace health research falls into this category. Examples of observational studies are case-controlled and cohort studies.

Case-controlled studies

Here researchers use existing records to identify people with a certain health problem ("cases") and a similar group without the problem ("controls").

For example, to learn whether a certain drug causes birth defects, one might collect data about children with defects (cases) and about those without defects (controls). The data are compared to see whether cases are more likely than controls to have mothers who took the drug during pregnancy. The case-controlled study may be the only way researchers can explore certain questions.

For example, it would be unethical to design a randomised controlled study deliberately exposing workers to a potentially harmful situation.

Cohort studies

For research purposes, a cohort is any group of people who are linked in some way and followed over time.

Researchers observe what happens to one group that has been exposed to a particular variable, for example, the effect of company downsizing on the health of office workers.

This group is then compared to a similar group that has not been exposed to the variable.

Experimental studies

Here researchers introduce an intervention and study the effects. Experimental studies are usually randomised, meaning the subjects are grouped by chance.

While not all controlled studies are randomised, all randomised trials are controlled. Another example of experimental studies, besides the Randomised controlled trial, is the controlled clinical trial.

Randomised controlled trials (RCT)

The randomised controlled trial is one of the simplest and most powerful tools of research. Simply put, the RCT is a study in which people are selected at random to receive one of several clinical interventions.

The participants in the RCT are defined as the study population (or subjects). Participants in the RCT are not necessarily ill, since the study can be conducted in healthy volunteers, in relatives of patients, or in members of the general public. The doctors who administer the interventions are called the investigators.

The interventions are also called clinical manoeuvres, and include actions of preventive strategies, diagnostic tests, screening programmes and treatments. For example, in a study where patients with a specific disease or condition are randomised to receive either a known or a new test drug.

Normally, a RCT measures and compares different events that are present or absent after the participants receive the interventions. These events are called outcomes. The RCT is regarded as a quantitative study since the outcomes are measured.

Controlled Clinical Trial (CCT)

This is similar to an RCT, except that subjects are not randomly assigned to the treatment or control groups. This increases the chance for bias, i.e., that people with similar qualities ended up in each of the groups, which could influence the final results.

Planning and reporting research

There are many different types of documents, protocols, reports and articles.

The research protocol

A research protocol is the legal document that outlines the study plan for a clinical trial. The plan must be carefully designed to safeguard the health and safety of the participants, as well as answer specific research questions.

A protocol describes who the participants are in the study; the schedule of tests, procedures, medications, dosage, and the length of the study.

While enrolled in a clinical trial, participants following a protocol are seen regularly by the research staff to monitor their health and to determine the safety and effectiveness of their treatment.

New Drug Application (NDA)

Following the completion of phase 3 clinical trials, a company analyses all the data, and if the data successfully demonstrates both safety and effectiveness, files an NDA with the authorities in each area (e.g. EU) where permission to market the drug is wanted.

The NDA contains all the scientific information that the company has gathered.

Approval for a new drug to be made widely available to the health care market typically takes about 12 - 18 months.

The authorities will review research data amounting to many thousands of pages. They will also weigh the need for a new drug when they evaluate each particular application.

A drug may qualify for fast-track review if it is designed to treat a life-threatening disease for which there are few alternative therapies.

Once the authorities approve the application, the new medicine can be made available for physicians to prescribe.

Discovering and developing a safe and effective new drug is a long, difficult, and expensive process, but once approved provides many benefits.

Besides abstracts and articles for peer reviewed journals (described below), there are many different types of documents, protocols and reports that you need to know about, e.g. clinical study reports, investigator brochures, package inserts, NDAs, IND filings and annual IND reports, DSMB reports, PSURs, etc.

No matter which type of document you are about to write, before you start writing, you should consider asking yourself the following general questions:

- What is the overall message that I want to communicate, and to whom? It is important who you are communicating to and that you never lose sight of your audience
- What information do I want to communicate, and what should I exclude? The more irrelevant information you communicate, the less effective your message will be
- What image do I want to project?
- How do I combine all of the above?
- How will my message be received, i.e. how will an editor treat it, and does the editor understand the benefits to the target audience?

Writing for peer-review journals

If you are writing a scientific paper it should be clear that your research is of vital importance and should thus be read by the broadest audience possible.

The purpose of having a research paper published is to ensure that you communicate it in a clear and concise way to enable your audience to:

- Assess your observations and conclusions
- Replicate your methods and results
- Determine if your conclusions are correctly drawn from the gathered data.

The most valuable advice prior to getting started is probably to become familiar with the general structure of a scientific paper.

Each journal has its own instruction for authors but they are all similar. They usually include four parts:

Introduction

The introduction part answers "what question did you ask yourself?". To make it easier, you should ask yourself the following questions:

- What do I have to communicate?
- Is my message worth communicating?
- Which format should I use?
- Which audience should receive my information?
- Which journal should I choose for my message?

Material and methods

This answers "what (e.g. subjects) was included and how was it studied?". Try to answer the following questions:

- How was the study designed, i.e. was it a randomised controlled study?
- How was it carried out, i.e. how were subjects included and how were they measured?
- How did you analyse the data and why did you choose this method?

- Can your research be easily replicated by others?

Results

This answers "What was discovered?". Here you report only the results of your investigation that are direct answers to the questions that you asked in the introduction section.

It is thus rather easy to write since the introduction part has helped you ask the right question, and the methods section has provided you with the means to answer it. To present the results optimally, ask yourself the following questions:

- Have I kept the results section as brief as possible?
- Is it clear and without my interpretations of the results?
- Have I resisted using references in this section?
- Does it contain text that tell the whole story, tables that summarise the results, illustrations that show the main results, and statistics that support the statements?

Discussion

This answers "What does the discovery mean?". This section is the most difficult one where you need to think, "So what?", i.e. why is my research interesting, relevant and how is it different from that of others? To get started, ask yourself the following questions:

- Have I summarised the relevant literature?
- What is currently known about the subject?
- How do my results add value?
- What is missing from the current knowledge, i.e. what needs further investigation?

References

When it comes to the style and how to present references I strongly suggest using a reference tool such as EndNote or Reference Manager.

When you are ready to submit your manuscript to the selected journal you should format it according to the instruction for authors.

Unless the reference format is already available through the reference tool it can often be downloaded from the journal homepage.

9 STATISTICS AND NUMBERS IN RESEARCH

Understanding basic statistical concepts is central to understanding the medical literature and it is not so important to understand the basis of the tests or the underlying mathematics.

You do, however, need to understand when a specific test should be used and how to interpret its results.

It is not complex or difficult – it actually helps you communicate your research effectively and accurately! Ask yourself the following questions about what you want to do:

- Do I want to describe a sample or outcome?
- Am I looking at how groups differ?
- Am I looking at how outcomes are related?
- Am I looking at changes over time?
- How should I measure my outcome?
- How is my outcome distributed in the sample?

The bad news is that you cannot engage in research and not understand how to use statistics. It is like cycling on a bike without wheels.

The good news is that you do not need to know everything.

Here are some of the essential parts of statistics that you need to know to be able to present your research (and to understand other's research), but it is explained in an easy and understandable way.

Only the most frequently used statistics is presented. Other more comprehensive books will present statistics in depth.

There are essentially three types of statistics in medical research:

- Descriptive statistics: numbers used to describe a sample, which does not test a hypothesis (for example, "mean" and "median")

- Parametric statistics: a very important statistic tool where you make sure that your data meets the assumptions (parameters) before the tests are performed (for instance, normality). Parametric data is continuous data, which is normally distributed.

- Non-parametric statistics: used for categorical, ordinal or non-normally distributed continuous data. It may check both parametric and non-parametric tests for congruity.

Most non-parametric tests are based on ranks or other non-value related methods. The interpretation answers if the P value is significant.

Percentage

Percentage means "per cent", which is Latin for "per hundred", describing a proportion of one hundred. 25% is 25 out of one hundred, or ¼ (75% is the same as ¾).

Percent is calculated by dividing the required number by the total (for example, 16 of the 50 students had salad for lunch. How many percent had salad? 16 divided by 50 equals to 0.32 which is 32%).

Incidence

The incidence describes the number of new cases of a condition over a given time. It is presented as a percentage of a population.

Prevalence

The prevalence describes the current amount of cases of a condition at a given time. It is, like the incidence, presented as a percentage of the studied population.

Mean

The mean is the same as the average and is the sum of the values divided by the number of values (for example, what is the mean height of boys in an school class? There are 8 boys with the following heights: 135 cm, 142 cm, 151cm, 135cm, 144cm, 139cm, 148cm and 150cm.

The mean is calculated by the total sum of cm divided by the amount of boys, i.e. 1144 divided by 8 equals to the 143cm).

Mean is used when your data is similar on both sides of the middle. This is called normal distribution, which means that the distribution of the data is pretty much bell-shaped, where the data on both sides of the middle appears similar.

Median

The median is the same as the mid-point and is used to represent the average where the data are not normally distributed (see mean), and is not presented like a bell-shaped curve. In a median, half of the values presented above and the other half below.

Standard deviation

Standard deviation (SD) is used for normally distributed data (see under mean). It describes how much the data varies around the mean (average) value, i.e. how much a set of values is spread around the average. SD should only be used when the data is normally distributed.

A range of one SD (i.e. ± 1 SD) above and below the average includes 68.2% of the data, while ± 2 SD includes 95.4%, and ± 3 SD includes 99.7% of the data.

Confidence interval

Confidence intervals (CI) are used to calculate a range (interval) where we can be pretty sure (confident) that the true value lies.

The CI is typically used when we, not only, need the average value of a sample, but we also need to know that a true population value is most likely to be included in the range.

If we, for example, would like to find out how many people in the UK suffer from allergy, we will need to take a sample of the population and calculate the mean from the sample.

This will, however, only provide us with the mean value in our specific sample of the population. If we take another sample of the population it will not give us the exact same value because many aspects can alter the results.

Therefore the CI gives us the range in which the true value is likely to be, i.e. the mean number of people with allergy if we were to study everyone in the UK.

P – value

The P - value, or probability value, is used when we want to show how likely it is that a hypothesis is true, where the hypothesis usually is, and that there is no difference between the two groups (the so called null-hypothesis).

The P - value gives the probability if the observed difference has occurred by chance.

If the P - value equals to 0.5 ($P = 0.5$) it means the probability that the difference has happened by chance is 0.5 (out of 1), i.e. 50:50 chance, but if $P = 0.05$ the probability that it happened by chance is 0.05 in 1, i.e. 1 in 20.

A P - value is significant if it is $P = 0.05$, highly significant if it is $P = 0.01$ (where the difference has happened by chance in 1 in 100), and very highly significant if it is $P = 0.001$ (where the difference has happened by chance in 1 in 1000).

Parametric test

Parametric tests are used to compare samples of data that is normally distributed. The most frequently used parametric test is the t test (or Student's t test). Other common parametric tests are X2 and analysis of variance (ANOVA).

Non-parametric tests

Non-parametric tests are used to compare samples of data that are not normally distributed. Instead of comparing the values, the data is ranked and then the ranks are compared.

The most commonly used nonparametric test is the Mann-Whitney U test.

Correlation and regression

In a situation where there is a linear relationship between two variables there is a correlation between them. A positive correlation means that both variables are increasing.

Smoking and cancer have a positive correlation since the more you smoke the greater the risk of cancer.

A negative correlation means that one variable goes up while the other goes down. Increased age and loss of vision have negative correlation since age increases while normal vision deteriorates.

Correlation is easily confused with regression. Regression is used to figure out how two different sets of data relates to each other.

Correlation, however, determines the strength of the association between variables whereas regression quantifies the association between them.

10 REFERENCES AND CITING

So, how do we secure that what we are communicating is correct?
Referencing is a standardised way of acknowledging the sources of
information and ideas that you have used in your assignments and it allows
the sources to be identified. It is important to be consistent when you are
referencing.

It is strongly suggested that everyone writing and citing medical information
invest in a reference handling software, e.g. EndNote or Reference
Manager. They offer a very user-friendly way of structuring and using
references.

It will also automatically format in-text citations and reference lists
according to the requirements of the journal, book etc. where your text will
be presented.

The software will ensure that no matter which output format you chose for
your citations and references, they are always presented according to the
Vancouver Style requirement. The Vancouver Style is a set if international
rules ensuring that citations and references are presented according to the
medical and ethical requirements. References presented according to the
Vancouver Style must:

- Record the full bibliographic details and relevant page numbers of the
  source from which information is taken

- Punctuation marks and spaces in the reference list and citations are very
  important

- Follow the punctuation and spacing exactly

- Insert the citation at the appropriate place in the text of your document

- Include a reference list that includes all in-text citations at the end of
  your document.

It is always important to accurately cite references in medical/scientific texts to acknowledge the sources. Science moves forward rapidly by knowledge, knowledge sharing, and further developing the work of others.

It is also important to reveal that you are familiar with the appropriate and relevant background knowledge to draw conclusions from the information you are working with.

Bluntly, are you clearly showing that you have done your homework, and are you thoroughly aware of the background and context into which your work fits? If yes, this is what gives you the permission to provide conclusions about the results you are presenting.

Reference citations also provide guidance for your audience to dig deeper in your specific subject and further follow up on your work.

Sources that need to be acknowledged are not limited to books and journal articles, but also include internet sites, computer software, written and e-mail correspondence, even verbal conversations with other people (in person or by telephone).

Therefore, you always need to clearly substantiate each statements by citing the original souses. The same goes for using figures, illustrations, or graphical material, either directly or in modified form.

Citing a statement as "common knowledge" is not enough – common knowledge always originates from someone or something. If you are in doubt, leave it out!

11 QUALITY CONTROL

Checking your work, or having it checked by someone else, before you submit the final text is crucial.

Everybody, including the most experienced writers, make mistakes and typos that may negatively influence the reader if left unidentified and uncorrected.

After working with your text from start to finish you need someone else to edit it, even if you have excellent editorial and proofreading skills.

Editing other writer's texts will also make you better at identifying improvable parts of your own material. Your text must be presented to your reader in the same way a new car is presented to a potential buyer.

The editor will help improve the text and flow by correcting punctuation, grammar and spelling errors in the same way the car salesman will wax, polish and finetune the car to make it look great in the eyes of the buyer.

Careful editing will significantly improve your text and thus help you accomplish the purpose with your message. Good editing includes reading the text out loud.

This stimulates both your vision and hearing. The more senses you stimulate the better the chance of catching potential errors.

Reading and editing from the beginning of your text often makes you think of new ideas to improve the message rather than focusing on editing for mistakes.

Therefore, read the sentences from back to front starting at the end of your text, through each paragraph toward the headings.

By reading one sentence at a time from the end you will find that the sentences still make sense but since it is being read differently you will focus more on errors and are less likely to wander away and start rewriting.

Always keep your dictionary handy to check the spelling, usage, and meanings of words if you are in doubt.

Alow your computer spell-checker to find errors but remember that it will only mark unrecognised words.

The spell-checker will thus not alert if you have left out words or if you are using words that may be correctly spelled but have incorrect meanings, for instance affect and effect.

Proofread the final draft more than one time. Let the text rest for a day or so before you proofread it again.

Reading the text with fresh eyes will sharpen your senses and increase the oportunity of finding possible errors. Even the most minor typing errors may alter the meaning of your text.

Make sure that you format text according the audience of the message. If you are preparing a manuscript for a medical journal, check the instructions for authors.

Such innstructions are almost always very clearly presented about what is expected and how it should be structured. Asking yourself the following questions is useful when you edit and profread your own and other author's texts:

- Have I provided a main idea or topic informing the reader of my purpose and focus?

- Have I provided the relevant details supporting my message?

- Have I presented the information in the correct order of importance?

- Have I structured the message according to the reader's needs?

- Have I structured sentences and paragraphs so according to the general flow of ideas?

- Have I presented sentences as active voice and are the paragraphs in a logical order?

- Have I presented the language in a clear, precise and suitable level to the reader?

- Have I eliminated repetition of ideas and unnecessary scientific or technical jargon?

- Have I presented anything that may be misunderstood or misinterpreted by the reader?

- Have I presented the text in an appropriate tone of voice?

- Have I presented any additional information that should be placed in an appendix?

- Have I cited sources where relevant, and have I presented the references correctly?

- Have I carefully proofread the text for spelling, grammar, punctuation, and flow?

12 SUMMARY AND FINAL ADVICE

This is the take home message, no matter what you are writing:

Plan your work

Spend lots of time brainstorming about what you want to communicate. Spend time doing your homework about the topic and all potential perspectives your message may contain.

Know your audience

Do not start writing until you have figured out who you are writing for. Who is your audience? What do they know? What do they need to know? What do they expect? What should you communicate to ensure the best possible effect of you message? How can you communicate the message to them? When should they receive the message? These are a few questions you must ask yourself!

Editing and proof-reading

Let your draft text rest a few days before you do a final proof-reading, or better yet, let someone else read it. Texts that you revise over a period of a few days will end up clearer and better organised.

Rather than edit your rough draft immediately after writing it, allow the text to rest a few days before returning to it. You will then have a better idea of how well you communicated your message.

Editing your paper will always improve your text. Your message may be more effective if you change paragraph order and condense some of your main points.

Formal or informal explanations

Always have your audience in mind, and make sure that you know what they want, expect and need. The people reading your message will probably not understand private jokes.

Informal terms and language may only confuse them. Take the time and make sure to explain fully every statement, reference and idea you present.

Active voice

Use active tense as much as possible since fewer words will make your message stronger. Use strong, concise, and clear language.

Do not repeat statements you have already communicated unless you are adding a new concept to the message.

Simple words

Instead of finding big, impressive words use simpler ones that are clear, precise, and convey your true meaning. The simpler you write the easier it is for your audience to understand what you are attempting to communicate.

Short words can be very effective, whereas the long complicated ones may cause confusion!

Software

Although the computer you use may catch spelling and grammar errors, never rely on it. Your software may automatically change words since it does not understand what you are communicating.

Read your draft text carefully and make sure you edit words to what you want them to be. This will minimise the risks of making embarrassing spelling and grammatical errors.

So, let us get started – and have lots of fun and success!

13 ADDITIONAL INFORMATION AND READING

Links, references and suggested reading:

European Medicines Agency (EMA), National competent authorities.

US Food and Drug Administration (FDA), Advertising Guidelines.

Stuart MC. The Complete Guide to Medical Writing. 2007.

Hall GM. How to write a paper. 2003.

Piantadosi S. Clinical Trials: A Methodologic Perspective Second Edition (Wiley Series in Probability and Statistics). 2005.

Goodman NW, Edwards MB and Black A. Medical Writing: A Prescription for Clarity. 2006.

Sahajwalla C. New Drug Development: Regulatory Paradigms for Clinical Pharmacology and Biopharmaceutics. 2004.

Pieterse H, Duijst P and de Jong MG. International Medical Device Clinical Investigations: A Practical Approach. 1999.

Emanuel EJ, Crouch RA, Arras JD and Moreno JD. Ethical and Regulatory Aspects of Clinical Research. 2003.

Machin D, Day S, Green S and Everitt BS. Textbook of Clinical Trials. 2004.

Soanes C and Stevenson A. Concise Oxford English Dictionary. 2008.

Cambridge Advanced Learner's Dictionary. 2005.

Chernecky CC and Berger BJ. Laboratory Tests and Diagnostic Procedures. 2007.

14 APPENDIX

List of common abbreviations

Ab	antibody
ADME	absorption, distribution, metabolism, excretion
ADR	adverse drug reaction
AE	adverse event
ANA	antinuclear antibody
ANCOVA	analysis of covariance
ANOVA	analysis of variance
AOB	any other business
AOC	area over the curve
ASAP	as soon as possible
assn.	association
asst.	assistant
ATC	anatomical therapeutic chemical
AUC	area under the curve
BCS	biopharmaceutical classification system
BG	blood glucose
BID	twice daily (bis in die)
BMI	body mass index
BSA	body surface area
BSE	bovine spongiform encephalopathy
BUN	blood urea nitrogen
CAPD	continuous ambulatory peritoneal dialysis
CATS	Cross-Application Time Sheet (time registration system)
CBER	Center for Biologics Evaluation and Research
CCDS	Company Core Data Sheet
CDC	Clinical Development Centre
CDER	Center for Drug Evaluation and Research
CDP	clinical development plan
CDT	clinical development team
CDW	Clinical Data Warehouse
CEO	chief executive officer
CFO	chief financial officer

CFR	Code of Federal Regulations (American legal code)
CGM	continuous glucose measurement
CHMP	Committee for Medicinal Products for Human Use
CI	confidence interval
CL/f	fractional clearance
Cmax	maximum concentration
CMC	Chemistry, Manufacturing and Control
CNS	central nervous system
Corp	Corporation
CPMP	Committee for Proprietary Medicinal Products (now CHMP)
CPoC	clinical proof of concept
CPS	clinical pharmacology scientist
CQA	clinical quality assurance
CRA	clinical research associate
CRD	Clinical Research Department
CRF	case report form
CRF	chronic renal failure
CRO	contract research organisation
CRP	C-reactive protein
CSF	critical success factor
CSO	chief scientific officer
CSR	clinical study report (ICH term)
CT	clinical trial
CTA	clinical trial application
CTA	clinical trial assistant
CTCAE	common terminology criteria for adverse events
CTD	common technical document
CTL	Clinical Trial Logistics
CTLA4	cytotoxic T-lymphocyte antigen 4
CTN	clinical trial notification
CTR	clinical trial report
CTS	Clinical Trial Safety
CV	curriculum vitae
CVI	corporate visual identity
CVP	corporate vice president
DB	database
DBL	database lock
DBR	database release
DC	dendritic cell
DCF	data clarification form
DHR	data handling report
DIA	Drug Information Association
DLQI	dermatology–life quality index

DM	Data Management
DMARDs	disease-modifying antirheumatic drugs
DNA	deoxyribonucleic acid
Dr	doctor
DRF	dose-range-finding
DRP	document-responsible person
EC	ethics committee
ECG	electrocardiograph
eCRF	electronic case report form
eCTD	electronic common technical document (electronic submission)
EDC	electronic data capture
EDM	electronic document management
ELISA	enzyme-linked immunosorbent assay
EMEA	European Medicines Agency
EOT	end of text (tables or figures)
EPAR	European Public Assessment Report
ESR	erythrocyte sedimentation rate
ESRD	end-stage renal disease
eTMF	electronic trial master file
EU	European Union
EVP	executive vice president
FAQ	frequently asked questions
FBG	fasting blood glucose
FDA	Food and Drug Administration
FHD	first human dose
FLS	fibroblast-like synoviocytes
FPFV	first patient first visit
FPG	fasting plasma glucose
FTE	full-time equivalent (employee)
GCP	Good Clinical Practice
GLP	Good Laboratory Practice
GMP	Good Manufacturing Practice
GxP	Good "anything" Practice
GH	growth hormone
GLP	Good Laboratory Practice
GMP	Good Manufacturing Practice
GPP	Good Pharmacoepidemiology Practice
GP	general practitioner
HA	health authority
HbA_{1c}	glycosylated haemoglobin
HCP	host cell protein

HDL	high-density lipoprotein
HE/OR	Health Economics/Outcomes Research
hGH	human growth hormone
HLA	human leukocyte antigen
HMWP	high molecular weight protein
HOMA	homeostatic model assessment
HR	Human Resources
HRQL	health-related quality of life
HRT	hormone replacement therapy
IB	investigator's brochure
IBD	inflammatory bowel disease
ICH	International Conference on Harmonisation
ICMJE	International Committee of Medical Journal Editors
IDB	integrated database
IDF	International Diabetes Foundation
IEC	independent ethics committee
IFN	interferon
IFNα	interferon alpha
IFNAR	interferon alpha receptor
Ig	immunoglobulin
IL	interleukin
i.m.	intramuscular
IMPACT	electronic trial steering system
IMPD	investigational medicinal product dossier
Inc	Incorporated
IND	investigational new drug
IRB	institutional review board (U.S. ethics committee)
ISE	integrated summary of efficacy
ISO	International Organization for Standardization
ISS	integrated summary of safety
IT	information technology
ITM	international trial manager
ITT	intention to treat
IU	international unit
i.v.	intravenous(ly)
J	journal
kg	kilogram
KO/KI	knock-out/knock-in
KPI	key performance indicator
L	litre
lb	pound

LLOQ	lower limit of quantification
LN	lupus nephritis
LOCF	last observation carried forward
LPFV	last patient first visit
LPLV	last patient last visit
LS	least squares
LSAD	low serum albumin in dialysis
LSFV/LV	last subject first visit/last visit
Ltd	Limited
LTR	Local Trials Registry
MAA	Marketing Authorisation Application
mAb	monoclonal antibody
MABEL	minimum anticipated biological effect level
MACE	major adverse cardiovascular event
MAS	macrophage inhibitory factor
MCP-1	monocyte chemotactic protein-1
MD	medical doctor
MD	multiple dose
MedDRA	Medical Dictionary for Regulatory Activities
MESI	medical event of special interest
mgmt	management
MHC	major histocompatibility complex
MIF	macrophage inhibitory factor
mL	millilitre
mm	millimetre
MMP	matrix metalloproteinase
Mr	Mister
MRI	magnetic resonance imaging
mRNA	messenger ribonucleic acid
MSA	master service agreement
MSc	Master of Science
MTD	maximum tolerated dose
MTX	methotrexate
MW	medical writer
NBE	new biologic entity
NCE	new chemical entity
NDA	new drug application
NICE	National Institute for Clinical Excellence
NK cells	natural killer cells
NMP	N-methyl-pyrrolidon
NOAEL	no observed adverse effect level
NPG	nocturnal plasma glucose
NSAIDs	nonsteroidal anti-inflammatory drugs

NTF	note to file
OAD	oral antidiabetic drug
OC	active osteoclasts
OTC	over-the-counter
PACT	public access to clinical trials
PASI	psoriasis area-and-severity index
PBMC	peripheral blood mononuclear cell
PD	pharmacodynamics
PDF	portable document format
PG	plasma glucose
PGA	physician's global assessment
PhD	Doctor of Philosophy
PI	package insert
PI	principal investigator
PK	pharmacokinetics (treat as singular)
PP	per protocol
PPG	postprandial glucose
PPPG	postprandial plasma glucose
Prof.	Professor
PsO	psoriasis
PSUR	periodic safety update report
PTF	peak-to-trough
PVP	project vice president
QA	quality assurance
QAP	quality activity plan
QC	quality control
QMR	quality management review
QMS	quality management system
QOL	quality of life
RA	Regulatory Affairs
RA	rheumatoid arthritis
RBC	red blood cell
RD	Research and Development
RTX	rituximab
Rx	medical prescription
SAE	serious adverse event
s.c.	subcutaneous(ly)
SD	single dose
SD	standard deviation
SDS	standard deviation score

SE	standard error
SEM	standard error of the mean
SGA	small for gestational age
SLA	service level agreement
SLE	systemic lupus erythematosus
SMFPG	self-measured fasting plasma glucose
SMPG	self-measured plasma glucose
SMQ	standardised MedDRA query
SOC	system organ class
SOP	standard operating procedure
SmPC	summary of product characteristics
SPC	supplementary patent certificate
STF	standard file
SU	sulphonylurea
$t\frac{1}{2}$	terminal half-life
T1DM	type 1 diabetes mellitus
T2DM	type 2 diabetes mellitus
TA	therapeutic area
TBA	to be announced
TBD	to be decided
TEAE	treatment-emergent adverse event
tel	telephone
TID	thrice daily (ter in die)
TM	trial manager/trial management
tmax	time to maximum concentration
TMF	trial master file
TNF-α	tumour necrosis factor alpha
TOC	table of contents
TVP	trial validation plan
ULN	upper limit of normal
UNR	upper normal range
U.K.	United Kingdom
VAS	visual analogue scale
VLDL-C	very low-density lipoprotein- cholesterol
WBC	white blood cells
WHO	World Health Organisation
WHO-ARD	World Health Organisation Adverse Reaction Dictionary

List of normal lab values and results

Red blood cells

RBC (Male)	4.2–5.6 M/μL
RBC (Female)	3.8–5.1 M/μL
RBC (Child)	3.5–5.0 M/μL

White Blood Cells

WBC (Male)	3.8–11.0 K / mm cubed
WBC (Female)	3.8–11.0 K / mm cubed
WBC (Child)	5.0–10.0 K / mm cubed

Haemoglobin

Hgb (Male)	14–18 g/dL
Hgb (Female)	11–16 g/dL
Hgb (Child)	10–14 g/dL
Hgb (Newborn)	15–25 g/dL

Hematocrit

Hct (Male)	39–54%
Hct (Female)	34–47%
Hct (Child)	30–42%
MCV	78–98 fL
MCH	27–35 pg
MCHC	31–37%
Neutrophils	50–81%
Bands	1–5%
Lymphocytes	14–44%
Monocytes	2–6%
Eosinophils	1–5%
Basophils	0–1%

Cardiac markers

Troponin I	0–0.1 ng/ml
Troponin T	0–0.2 ng/ml
Myoglobin (Male)	10–95 ng/ml
Myoglobin (Female)	10–65 ng/ml

BNP	Greater than 500 pg/ml (suggesting congestive hear failure)
BNP	Less than 100 pg/ml (unlikely congestive heart failure)
CK-MB	0−3.9%

Ejection fraction

55-70%	Normal
40-55%	mild LV dysfunction
30-40%	moderate LV dysfunction
<30%	severe LV dysfunction

General chemistry

Acetone	0.3−2.0 mg%
Albumin	3.5−5.0 gm/dL
Alkaline Phosphatase	32−110 U/L
Ammonia	11−35 μmol/L
Amylase	50−150 U/dL
Anion gap	5−16 mEq/L
AST, SGOT (Male)	7−21 U/L
AST, SGOT (Female)	6−18 U/L
direct bilirubin	0−0.4 mg/dL
indirect bilirubin	total bilirubin minus direct bilirubin
total bilirubin	0.2−1.4 mg/dL
BUN	6−23 mg/dL
Calcium (total)	8−11 mg/dL
Carbon dioxide	21−34 mEq/L
Chloride	96−112 mEq/L
Creatinine	0.6−1.5 mg/dL
Ethanol	0 mg% ; Coma: greater than or equal to 400−500 mg%
ferritin	13−300 ng/mL
GGT (male)	11−63 IU/L
GGT (female)	8−35 IU/L
folic acid	2.0−21 ng/mL
Glucose	70−110 mg/dL
HbA1c	4−6% is normal (diabetic patients are to keep the value <7-8%)
Iron	52−169 μg/dL
Iron binding capacity	246−455 μg/dL
Lactic acid	0.4−2.3 mEq/L

Lactate	0.3–2.3 mEq/L
LDH	56–194 IU/L
Lipase	10–140 U/L
Magnesium	1.5–2.5 mg/dL
Osmolarity	276–295 mOsm/kg
parathyroid hormone	12–68 pg/mL
Phosphorus	2.2–4.8 mg/dL
Potassium	3.5 - 5.5 mEq/L
Protein (total)	6.0–9.0 gm/dL
SGPT	8–32 U/L
Sodium	135–148 mEq/L
T3	0.8–1.1 µg/dL
Thyroglobulin	Less than 55 ng/mL
Thyroxine (T4) total	5–13 µg/dL
Total protein	5–9 gm/dL
TSH	Less than 9 µU/mL
Urea nitrogen	8–25 mg/dL
Uric acid (Male)	3.5–7.7 mg/dL
Uric acid (Female)	2.5–6.6 mg/dL

Lipids (adults)

Cholesterol (total)	Less than 200 mg/dL
Cholesterol (HDL)	30–75 mg/dL
Cholesterol (LDL)	Less than 130 mg/dL
Triglycerides (Male)	Greater than 40–170 mg/dL
Triglycerides (Female)	Greater than 35–135 mg/dL

Urinalysis

Color	Straw
specific gravity	1.003–1.040
pH	4.6–8.0
sodium	10–40 mEq/L
potassium	Less than 8 mEq/L
chloride	Less than 8 mEq/L
protein	1–15 mg/dL
rbc's	0–2 per hpf
wbc's	0–2 per hpf
ketones	negative
blood	negative
urobilogen	0.2–1.0 Ehr U/dl
urine nitrite	negative

osmolality   80–1300 mOsm/L

24-hour urine

amylase   250 –1100 IU/24 hr
calcium   100–250 mg/24 hr
chloride   110–250 mEq/24 hr
creatinine   1–2 g/24 hr
creatine clearance ()   100 - 140 mL/min
creatine clearance (♂)   16–26 mg/kg/24 hr
creatine clearance (ʏ)   80–130 mL/min
creatine clearance (ʏ)   10–20 mg/kg/24 hr
magnesium   6–9 mEq/24 hr
osmolality   450–900 mOsm/kg
phosphorus   0.9–1.3 g/24 hr
potassium   35–85 mEq/24 hr
protein   0–150 mg/24 hr
sodium   30–280 mEq/24 hr
urea nitrogen   10–22 gm/24 hr
uric acid   240–755 mg/24 hr

Coagulation

ACT   90–130 seconds
APTT   21–35 seconds
Platelets   140 000–450 000/mL
Plasminogen   62–130%
PT   10–14 seconds
PTT   32–45 seconds
FSP   Less than 10 µg/dL
fibrinogen   160–450 mg/dL
bleeding time   3–7 minutes
thrombin time   11–15 seconds

Cerebrospinal fluid

appearance   clear
glucose   40–85 mg/dL
osmolality   290–298 mOsm/L
pressure   70–180 mm/H2O

99

protein	15–45 mg/dL
total cell count	0–5 cells
wbc's	0–6/μL

Neurological values

| cerebral perfusion pressure | 70–90 mm Hg |
| intracranial pressure | 5–15 mm Hg or 5 - 10 cm H2O |

Arterial values

pH	7.35–7.45
PCO2	35–45 mmHg
bicarbonate	22–26 mEq/L
O2 sat	96–100%
PO2	85–100 mmHg
base excess	-2 to +2 mmol/L

Venous values

pH	7.31–7.41
PCO2	41–51 mmHg
bicarbonate	22–29 mEq/L
O2 sat	60–85%
PO2	30–40 mmHg
base excess	0 to +4 mmol/L

Body Mass Index (BMI)

Underweight	<18.5
Normal weight	18.5–24.9
Overweight	25–29.9
Obesity	>30
Morbid Obesity	>40

ABOUT THE AUTHOR

Patrick Wulf Hanson is a dedicated scientific and medical communicator and project manager who has worked within the field of medicine/science and research in Denmark, Sweden and USA for over 20 years.

Patrick has always been able to concretely interpret and describe the most complicated inner workings of the human body and other scientific organisms in a simple and understandable way.

Patrick is often invited to evaluate complex medical and scientific topics where he takes pride in exploring and answering questions about the nature of complex scientific subjects.

Patrick spent six years in the pharmaceutical industry where he worked with both drugs and devices in Regulatory Affairs, Product Safety and Corporate Branding.

In his work, he has covered everything from planning and writing peer reviewed articles, newsletters, detailing and brochures for marketing to more complex medical translations and strategic global projects related to communication concepts with regulators and other authorities.

Patrick's experience also includes being responsible for developing and managing interdisciplinary medical information within all therapeutic areas as well as establishing contacts to the leading KOLs in all therapeutic areas.

This has further strengthened his medical and scientific knowledge and understanding. Besides publishing a number of peer review articles, as a scientist Patrick has also planned, developed and managed training courses, e-learning concepts and a large quantity of other forms of scientific projects.

www.ingramcontent.com/pod-product-compliance
Lightning Source LLC
Chambersburg PA
CBHW051334170526
45166CB00002B/810